MW00474311

Attention Deficit Hyperactivity Disorder
in Adults

The latest assessment and treatment strategies

Russell A. Barkley, PhD

Clinical Professor of Psychiatry
Medical University of South Carolina
Research Professor of Psychiatry
State University of New York Upstate Medical School

JONES AND BARTLETT PUBLISHERS
Sudbury, Massachusetts
BOSTON   TORONTO   LONDON   SINGAPORE

World Headquarters

Jones and Bartlett Publishers
40 Tall Pine Drive
Sudbury, MA 01776
978-443-5000
info@jbpub.com
www.jbpub.com

Jones and Bartlett Publishers
Canada
6339 Ormindale Way
Mississauga, Ontario L5V 1J2
Canada

Jones and Bartlett Publishers
International
Barb House, Barb Mews
London W6 7PA
United Kingdom

Jones and Bartlett's books and products are available through most bookstores and online booksellers. To contact Jones and Bartlett Publishers directly, call 800-832-0034, fax 978-443-8000, or visit our website www.jbpub.com.

Substantial discounts on bulk quantities of Jones and Bartlett's publications are available to corporations, professional associations, and other qualified organizations. For details and specific discount information, contact the special sales department at Jones and Bartlett via the above contact information or send an email to specialsales@jbpub.com.

The authors, editor, and publisher have made every effort to provide accurate information. However, they are not responsible for errors, omissions, or for any outcomes related to the use of the contents of this book and take no responsibility for the use of the products and procedures described. Treatments and side effects described in this book may not be applicable to all people; likewise, some people may require a dose or experience a side effect that is not described herein. Drugs and medical devices are discussed that may have limited availability controlled by the Food and Drug Administration (FDA) for use only in a research study or clinical trial. Research, clinical practice, and government regulations often change the accepted standard in this field. When consideration is being given to use of any drug in the clinical setting, the health care provider or reader is responsible for determining FDA status of the drug, reading the package insert, and reviewing prescribing information for the most up-to-date recommendations on dose, precautions, and contraindications, and determining the appropriate usage for the product. This is especially important in the case of drugs that are new or seldom used.

Production Credits

Publisher: Christopher Davis
Acquisitions Editor: Alison Hankey
Custom Projects Editor: Kathy Richardson
Production Editor: Wendy Swanson
Marketing Manager: Ilana Goddess
V.P., Manufacturing and Inventory Control: Therese Connell
Text Design: Coleridge Design
Composition: John Garland
Cover Design: Coleridge Design
Printing and Binding: Malloy, Inc.
Cover Printing: Malloy, Inc.

Library of Congress Cataloging-in-Publication Data

Barkley, Russell A., 1949–
Attention deficit hyperactivity disorder in adults : the latest assessment and treatment strategies / Russell A. Barkley.
    p. ; cm.
  Includes bibliographical references and index.
  ISBN 978-0-7637-6564-4 (pbk. : alk. paper)
  1. Attention deficit disorder in adults—Handbooks, manuals, etc. I. Title.
  [DNLM: 1. Attention Deficit Disorder with Hyperactivity—diagnosis—Handbooks. 2. Attention Deficit Disorder with Hyperactivity—therapy—Handbooks. 3. Adult. WM 34 B256a 2009]
  RC394.A85B38 2009
  616.85'89—dc22
                2008047749

6048

Printed in the United States of America
13 12 11 10   10 9 8 7 6 5 4 3 2

Read Me First

This book is orientated toward the practitioner, with easy-to-read treatment descriptions and examples. It is written in a nonacademic style and formatted to make the first reading, as well as ongoing reference, quick and easy. You will find:

▶ **Sidebars** — Narrow columns in the margin of each page highlight important information, preview upcoming sections or concepts, and define terms used in the text.

▶ **Definitions** — Terms are defined in the sidebars where they originally appear in the text and in an alphabetical glossary on pages 67 through 70.

▶ **References** — Numbered references appear in the text after information from those sources. Full references appear on pages 71 through 77.

▶ **Key Concepts** — At the end of each chapter, we include a review list of key concepts from that chapter. Use these lists for ongoing quick reference and for reviewing what you learned from reading the chapter.

Contents

Chapter One: Adult ADHD in Perspective   I

What Is ADHD and How Does It Affect Adult Patients? 1

    Health 3

    Relationship Problems 4

    Educational Achievement 5

    Employment 6

    Money 8

    Driving Safety 8

How Does ADHD Change Its Presentation Across the Lifespan? 9

What Causes ADHD? 12

    Genetics 12

    Other Factors 12

    The Neurobiology of ADHD 12

    Conclusion 13

Chapter Two: Diagnosis and Assessment   15

What Current Diagnostic Criteria Exist for ADHD? 15

How May Clinicians Best Use the *DSM-IV-TR* Diagnostic Criteria When Working with Adults? 17

What Problems Exist in Using the *DSM-IV-TR* Criteria with Adult Patients? 18

    Criteria Causing Concern in Adult ADHD Diagnosis 18

        Age of Onset 18

        Appropriateness of the Symptom List to Adults 19

        Threshold for Diagnosis 20

        Presentation of ADHD in Adults 20

        Degree of Impairment 20

    Challenges of Diagnosing ADHD in Adults 21

        Lack of Specificity 21

        Lack of Objective Quantitative Measures 21

        Malingering 22

        Under-Reporting of Impairment 22

Are There Better Criteria for Diagnosing Adult ADHD Than the Current *DSM-IV-TR* Criteria? 23

    Differential Diagnosis 24

Bipolar Disorder (BPD) 26

Substance Use and Abuse 27

Major Depression 27

Anxiety Disorders 28

Borderline Personality Disorder 28

Comorbidity 29

What Assessment Tools Help Diagnose Adult ADHD? 30

Structured Interviews 30

Adult ADHD Interview 30

Barkley's Quick Check for Adult ADHD Diagnosis 30

Structured Clinical Interview for DSM-IV (SCID) 30

Self-Reporting Scales 31

Adult ADHD Self-Report Scale (ASRS) 31

Adult ADHD Investigator Symptom Rating Scale (AISRS) 31

Barkley's Adult ADHD Quick Screen 31

Brown ADD Rating Scale 31

Conners' Adult Attention-Deficit Rating Scale (CAARS) 31

The Symptom Checklist 90—Revised 32

Wender Utah Rating Scale (WURS) 32

Archival Records 32

Neuropsychological Tests 33

Behavior Rating Inventory of Executive Function (BRIEF) 33

Conners' Continuous Performance Task or Test (CPT) 33

Stroop Word Color Test 34

Wechsler Adult Intelligence Scale, Third Edition (WAIS-III)—Digit Span Subtest

....34

Chapter Three: Pharmacological Treatment   **37**

What Medications Are Available to Treat ADHD? 37

Pharmacology of ADHD Stimulant Medications 38

FDA-Approved Medications for ADHD in Adults 39

Stimulant Medications 39

Dexmethylphenidate, Extended-Release 40

Lisdexamfetamine Dimesylate (LDX) 40

Methylphenidate, OROS Extended Release 41

Mixed Amphetamine Salts (MAS), Extended-Release 41

Nonstimulant Medications 42

Atomoxetine 42

Antidepressants 43

What Special Considerations Exist for Medication Treatment in Adults with ADHD? 44

Long- vs. Short-Acting Stimulant Medications 44

Medication Misuse and abuse 45

Contraindications and Adverse Events...................................45

Treatment of Comorbid Conditions 46

How Is ADHD Pharmacotherapy Managed?...............................46

Treatment Goals 48

Chapter Four: Nonpharmacological Treatment   51

What Are the Goals of Psychosocial Treatment of Adult ADHD?............51

What Psychosocial Treatments Are Available for Adults with ADHD?.........53

Psychoeducation 53

Cognitive-Behavioral Therapy (CBT).....................................54

Other Treatment Modalities for Adults with ADHD.......................57

Support Person...57

Couples Therapy..57

Group Therapy 58

What Unique Challenges Face Adults with ADHD? What Can Be Done to Help Adults with ADHD Cope with These Challenges? 59

Health 59

Sexual Health..59

Relationships and Child-Rearing 60

Education 61

College and Vocational Training......................................61

Employment 62

Personal Coaching 62

Vocational Counseling 63

General Strategies for Success at Work...............................63

Finances 64

Driving Safety 65

Glossary   67

References   71

Index   78

Chapter One:
Adult ADHD in Perspective

This chapter answers the following:

▶ **What Is ADHD and How Does It Affect Adult Patients?** —This section provides an overview of adult ADHD and outlines the domains in which ADHD affects the lives of adult patients, including health, education, work, relationships, finances, and driving safety.

▶ **How Does ADHD Change in Its Presentation Across the Lifespan?** —This section explains how ADHD symptoms change with a patient's age and focuses on the self-control problems unique to adults with ADHD.

▶ **What Causes ADHD?** —This section examines the influences of genetic factors, the most important cause of ADHD, as well as environmental biohazards that may cause ADHD. A brief overview of the contribution of brain structure and chemistry is provided.

A WARENESS and diagnosis of *attention deficit/hyperactivity disorder (ADHD) in adults* are growing rapidly. What was once considered a childhood disorder one could outgrow is now recognized as a disease that can span an individual's lifetime, resulting in considerable impairments. Adult ADHD research has come into its own recently, bringing hope for improved quality of life to millions of patients with previously undiagnosed cases.

What Is ADHD and How Does It Affect Adult Patients?

Attention deficit/hyperactivity disorder (ADHD) is a *neuropsychiatric disorder* that usually first becomes apparent in early childhood, when the child's functioning begins to be negatively impacted by *inattention, hyperactivity*, and *impulsivity*. ADHD symptoms persist across the lifespan, with estimates of 50%–65% of children with ADHD continuing to experience severe symptoms and related impairment into adulthood.[1] However, symptom patterns change as people with ADHD age. For example, while children with ADHD are more likely to exhibit problems with hyperactivity, adults with ADHD are more likely to demonstrate problems with inattention, *self-control*, organization, and time management.[1,2] Recent research indicates that 4.4% of the United States adult population has ADHD.[3] Based on United States Census 2000 population figures, approximately 9 million adults suffer from ADHD.[3,4]

Research shows that adults with ADHD suffer significant consequences and impairments in multiple life domains. Several of

attention deficit/hyperactivity disorder (ADHD) — a neuropsychiatric disorder that usually becomes apparent in early childhood. Its symptoms of hyperactivity, impulsivity, and/or inattention often persist across the lifespan

neuropsychiatric disorder — a behaviorial disorder characterized by structural and functional abnormalities of the nervous system

inattention — the state of being distracted, or the inability to concentrate; inattention by itself may result from a variety of physical and emotional conditions, including stress

hyperactivity — a state of heightened motor and emotional activity or excitability

impulsivity — a lack of self-control over one's actions and words; the inability to consider the consequences of actions and words before speaking or carrying out actions

self-control — ability to direct actions at oneself to change or restrain one's own behavior

UMass study — a recently completed, NIMH-funded study comparing (1) adults not diagnosed with ADHD who self-referred to an ADHD clinic with (2) a community control group and (3) a group of patients in the same clinic who had other psychiatric disorders

Milwaukee study — a recently completed, NIMH-funded study of children with ADHD diagnosis followed into adulthood (mean age 27), comparing adults who still met diagnostic criteria for ADHD with those who no longer met the criteria and with a community control group who never received an ADHD diagnosis.

comorbid disorder — a disease or condition occurring at the same time as another disease or condition, but which is unrelated to it

the more recent studies have focused on life outcomes for adults with ADHD. These include:[1, 5-7]

Studies funded by the National Institute of Mental Health (NIMH)—with results published in a book, *ADHD in Adults: What the Science Says*—evaluated two ADHD adult populations:

1. **The University of Massachusetts Medical School (the** *UMass study***)** compared a group of 146 adults who had self-referred to an ADHD clinic and who were eventually given an ADHD diagnosis with two control groups: (1) a clinical control group of 97 adults seen at the same clinic but who had a diagnosis of other psychiatric disorders, primarily anxiety disorders, and (2) a (healthy) community control group of 109 adults. The average age in these groups was between 32 and 38 years of age.[1]

2. **The Medical College of Wisconsin Study in Milwaukee (the** *Milwaukee study***)** evaluated adults who received an ADHD diagnosis in childhood and were followed into adulthood (mean age 27, age range 22–32). The Milwaukee study compared the following groups on numerous measures of life impairments:

   ▶ Adults who received a diagnosis of ADHD in childhood (hyperactive child syndrome, H) and still met diagnostic criteria for ADHD at a mean age of 27 (H+ADHD)

   ▶ Adults who received a diagnosis of ADHD in childhood but no longer met diagnostic criteria as adults at a mean age of 27 (H-ADHD)

   ▶ A community control group that had been monitored over the same time period

In both of these studies the ADHD and control groups were predominantly male and Caucasian. Additionally, the people in the ADHD groups, like most people with ADHD, suffered from a significant amount of *comorbid* conditions, including substance abuse or dependence, anxiety, and depression.[1]

Biederman et al. evaluated the perceptions of adults with ADHD regarding work and relationships among other items. Five hundred people with self-reported ADHD diagnoses were identified and interviewed from a US nationally representative digital phone sample. This population was age and gender matched to a group of 501 adults reporting that they did not have an ADHD diagnosis. The mean age of the ADHD group was 32 years and 49% of the population was male. Comorbidity with other mental health disorders was not reported.[5,6]

The World Health Organization sponsored a study of ADHD in adults in 10 world countries, including 3197 adults in the United

States. An ADHD diagnosis was confirmed by assessment scales and interviews including the Composit International Diagnostic Interview (CIDI), the ADHD Clinical Diagnostic Scale (ACDS), and the ADHD Rating Scale (ADHD-RS). Employment role performance was evaluated using the WHO-Disability Assessment Scale and the WHO Health and Work Performance Questionnaire. The age range was 18–44 years for the United States population with more males than females identified with ADHD. Comorbidity with other mental health disorders was not reported.[7]

These research studies support earlier findings on adults with ADHD and add substantial new information confirming the serious consequences of ADHD across multiple areas of patients' lives, including health, relationships, education, employment, and finances.[1,5-7]

Health

Adults with ADHD tend to be impulsive and have difficulty with paying attention, planning, managing time, and considering the consequences of their actions. These problems often result in poorer preventive health measures and self-care, which in turn may put adults with ADHD at greater risk for medical problems such as infections, cardiovascular disease, accidental injuries, and even early death. Recent research from the Milwaukee study shows that adults with ADHD have the following health and lifestyle risks and outcomes, compared to a control group:[1]

Behavioral patterns involving poor self-care may put the adult with ADHD at greater risk for medical problems such as infections, cardiovascular disease, cancer, accidental injuries, and even early death.

▶ **Heart disease** — 2.4 times higher Total Coronary Heart Disease points (risk)

▶ **Body mass index** — 11.4% higher

▶ **Cholesterol** — 16% lower HDL cholesterol, 20% higher ratio of total/HDL cholesterol

▶ **Nonmedical drug use** — 2.2 times more likely

▶ **Medical/dental problems** — 32% more concerns

▶ **Sleep problems** — 2.5 times more likely

These research results demonstrate that the risks and lifestyle problems listed above likely predispose adults with ADHD, compared with control groups, to:[1]

▶ More medical problems

▶ Increased use of the healthcare system (and greater associated costs)

▶ Increased use of sick days from employment

▶ More emotional disorders, antisocial activities, and substance use and abuse

Recent research also shows that, compared with control groups, adults with ADHD show increased high-risk behavior or mental disorders, such as:[1,3,8,9]

- ▶ **Tobacco use** — 2–3 times more likely[1,3,5]
- ▶ **Alcohol abuse or dependence problems** — 3–8 times more likely[1,3,8]
- ▶ **Drug abuse or dependence problems** — 3–8 times more likely[1,3,8]
- ▶ **Depression** — 3–6 times more likely[1,3,8]
- ▶ **Anxiety** — 8–17 times more likely[1,3,8]
- ▶ **Antisocial Personality Disorder or behavior**—1–4 times more likely[1,8]

Increased incidences of high-risk behaviors and mental disorders result in adults with ADHD being 1.5 to 2.5 times more likely to be arrested than age-matched controls.[1]

Adults with ADHD also tend to engage in higher risk sexual activity, a further complication of medical and psychological risks. While they do not exhibit a greater rate of sexual disorders than other adults, they have a history of more unprotected sex and more sexual partners over a 10-year period, compared to age-matched peer control groups. This puts adults with ADHD at ten times greater risk for teenage pregnancy and four times greater risk for sexually transmitted diseases (STDs) than those in control groups. Because of this high-risk sexual lifestyle, adults with ADHD get tested for HIV far more often than their peers. Fortunately, at this time, adults with ADHD do not seem to have a greater rate of HIV infection.[1,5,10]

Relationship Problems

In the Milwaukee study, more adults with ADHD professed to a lack of sexual desire "sometimes or more often" (49%) compared with 24% of controls and 25% of the H- group.

Intimacy, cohabitation, and marital function are also impaired in adults with ADHD. Research in 1992 found a relationship between adult ADHD and high rates of divorce and separation.[11] A small 2003 study also reported that marital and family functioning was more impaired in an adult ADHD group, compared with controls.[12]

Because ADHD has a strong genetic component (see The Neurobiology of ADHD section on pages 12–13), many adults with ADHD also have children affected by the disorder or by other challenging behavioral disorders, such as oppositional defiant disorder.

Adults with ADHD report less satisfying relationships with their marital or cohabiting partners[1,8,10] and, compared with age-matched peer control groups, they have double the divorce rate.[5] The 2003 study showed that a much higher proportion had affairs while married.[12] Adults with ADHD also tend to be more volatile and to report themselves as being likely to break up a relationship over trivial issues.[5,10]

Recent research found that 40% of adults[5] with diagnosed ADHD had children with significantly elevated symptoms of the disorder. The dual challenge of coping with both a partner's and a child's ADHD further strains relationships among couples.[1,12] In addition, due to risky sexual behavior (discussed above in "Health"), many adolescents and young adults with ADHD have children at a time of life when they are less prepared for the challenges of maintaining a healthy family life.

The UMass study found that adults with ADHD were less likely to have been married or to be currently married than adults in the community control group. This study, however, did not support a connection between adult ADHD and higher divorce rates, probably because of the young mean age of the participants (early 30s) and thus the limited duration of marriages. Additionally, ratings of marital satisfaction by spouses with ADHD tend to be significantly lower than the control group ratings, foreboding future increased risks of marital instability for those with ADHD.[1,5]

Recent research shows that adults with ADHD, compared to control groups, have:[1,5,8]

► 2 times more divorces

► 4 times more likely to have complaints of poor-quality relationships

► 4.6 times more likely to have extramarital affairs

► 2 times higher levels of parenting-related stress

This suggests that adults with ADHD are more likely to have significant interpersonal, cohabiting, and marital problems. In addition, they have more offspring morbidity and child management difficulties at clinical presentation than do adults in the general population.

Educational Achievement

Extensive historical research has documented pervasive educational problems for children with ADHD.[1,13,14] Inattentiveness, impulsivity, and/or hyperactivity cause most students with ADHD to underperform relative to their own abilities. For example, among students with ADHD:[1,5,8,14-19]

► Up to 56% require academic tutoring

► About 30% or more repeat a grade

► Thirty to forty percent require special education services

► Significantly fewer are likely to graduate from high school or college

► Significantly more receive grades of Cs or lower

By adolescence, ADHD symptoms tend to interfere with educational performance in more numerous and concrete ways. Research studies show that students with ADHD have significant problems as outlined in Table 1.1 on the following page.[1,9]

Table 1.1   Educational Performance of Students with and without ADHD[1,5,8,14]

Performance Measure	Students without ADHD (%)	Students with ADHD (%)
Failure of a grade	8–15	30–47
Suspension from school	18–21	60–71
Graduation from high school	93–99	62–83
Graduation from college	26–68	9–19

> *Students with ADHD are significantly more likely to have lower high school grade point averages than their peers without ADHD.*[1]

> *Scores obtained on standardized academic achievement tests by children with ADHD (90 to 95) average ½ to 1 standard deviation below the mean standard score of 100 obtained by counterparts without ADHD.*[17]

These studies indicate that ADHD diagnosed in childhood substantially impairs the educational achievement of those growing up with the disorder, whether or not they had retained the full disorder into adulthood.

Research has yielded conflicting results on ADHD's relationship to intelligence. Some research indicates that adults with ADHD have lower IQ scores on standardized tests,[8,20] which is similar to the results of numerous studies of children with the disorder. Other research finds no difference in intelligence in those with ADHD who self-refer to clinics.[21-23] Recent research shows that children with ADHD who grow into adults with ADHD have a 7- to 10-point lower intelligence estimate than their peers without ADHD, while clinic-referred adults with ADHD do not appear to have IQ scores different from the clinic's adults without ADHD.[21-23] This suggests a referral bias; adults who self-refer to clinics and receive a diagnosis of ADHD as adults have been shown to have higher intellectual levels than do adults who received a diagnosis of ADHD in childhood.[1] It appears that children living in a family with a variety of protective factors in place may cope better with the symptoms of ADHD, thus avoiding a diagnosis of ADHD during childhood. These protective factors may include high IQ; economic resources; good social skills; quality, individualized schooling; or a positive family environment.[24] However, the greater independence of adult individuals from their families and such protective factors, along with the greater complexities and stressors of the adult world, may lead adults with undiagnosed ADHD to become impaired and to seek treatment.

Employment

> *Adults with ADHD may prefer jobs and tasks that are varied and active, rather than routine, repetitive, and sedate.*

Adults with ADHD perform significantly worse in the workplace than their peers without ADHD.[1,5,14] In studies, employers rated these adults as less adequate in fulfilling work demands, less competent in performing their job duties, less likely to work independently and to complete tasks, and less likely to get along well with supervisors. Additionally, compared with their peers without ADHD, adults with ADHD tend to change jobs more frequently, get dismissed from jobs more frequently, work more part-time jobs, and report more often that certain tasks at work are too difficult.[1,5,10] Finally, they are less likely to be currently employed full time.[5,6]

A recent study by the World Health Organization concluded that the number of days of work lost by workers with ADHD in the United States was 10.1 days annually.[7] Another study estimated that the loss of workforce productivity in the US associated with ADHD in 2003 was between $67 billion and $116 billion.[6]

Overall, adults with ADHD have more employment difficulties than their peers without ADHD. Specifically, research shows that they have the following problem rates, compared with peers without ADHD:[1,3,5-7,10,14]

- ▶ **Job terminations** (firings) — 2–4 times higher rates[1,14]
- ▶ **Behavior problems on the job** — 19 times more[1]
- ▶ **Disciplinary actions in the workplace** — 18 times more[1]
- ▶ **Job changes** — 52% more[1]
- ▶ **Absenteeism and reduced role performance at work** — Average of 22 more days per year[3,7]
- ▶ **Average monthly income** — 20–40% less (and thus overall lower socioeconomic status)[1,3,5,6]

In addition, adults with ADHD show:

- ▶ More difficulty following instructions, getting along with coworkers, and meeting deadlines[1,5]
- ▶ More difficulty managing large workloads, concentrating, and paying attention[5]
- ▶ Lower job status and lower rates of professional employment[1,3,5]

In the workplace, adults with ADHD tend to be disorganized, miss deadlines, fail to keep commitments, lose track of important details, proceed on projects without first listening to directions, and have irritable and sometimes hostile relationships with coworkers. While many adults in general experience such problems on occasion, adults with ADHD do so far more frequently and with greater adverse impact on job performance than do others without the disorder.[1,3,5]

The best predictor of workplace performance in adults with ADHD appears to be the severity of their ADHD symptoms. In fact, the severity of self-reported ADHD symptoms, as well as employer ratings of the severity of ADHD in the workplace, significantly predicted lower ratings of workplace performance.[1]

Recent research found that 71% more adults with ADHD (compared to the control group) quit their jobs as a result of their own hostility toward others in the workplace.[1]

Money

The inattentive, distractible, and poorly inhibited behavior of adults with ADHD can impair their management of money and general financial status. Prior to the UMass and Milwaukee studies, however, no studies had examined this effect in detail. These studies found that impulsive buying and difficulties with self-regulation led to financial difficulties in adults with ADHD.[1] In 2001, research also found that adults with ADHD reported more frequent shopping sprees and more trouble sticking to a budget than did a control group.[10] Recent research shows that adults with ADHD earned less money, saved less money, and had problems managing money.[1,6] Specifically those with ADHD, compared to control group peers:

- ▶ Earn 20–40% less money[1,3,5,6]
- ▶ Save only $2 for every $10 that someone without ADHD saves[1]
- ▶ Have 4.5 times higher likelihood of having difficulty managing their money[1]
- ▶ Have 5.2 times higher risk of impulse-buying[1]
- ▶ Are 3.7 times more likely to have a poor credit rating[1,14]

Adults with ADHD in the UMass study were significantly more likely than community controls to have utilities turned off for nonpayment, miss a loan repayment, and exceed credit card limits. Many, in contrast to those in control groups, had not begun saving for retirement.[1] The UMass study clearly shows that, compared with those in the other two study groups, adults with ADHD are more likely to demonstrate difficulties with managing money at initial clinical presentation.[1]

Driving Safety

Multiple studies have found that of all possible causes of vehicular accidents, driver inattention is among the most common. This is especially so for in-vehicle distractions, such as talking to others, playing with the sound system, or using a cell phone. The combination of impulsive actions and *distractibility* related to ADHD makes it dangerous for adults with ADHD to get behind the wheel. Combined with slower and more variable reaction time and, in some cases, reduced motor speed and coordination, these symptoms of ADHD in a teen or adult can further predispose them to having significant problems operating a motor vehicle.[1,25]

The first study to report data on a possible connection between hyperactivity (i.e., ADHD) in children and increased driving risks in the teen and adult years was published in 1979.[26] Numerous studies in later years confirmed this association and

distractibility — stimuli in the environment attract attention away from the task at hand

greatly expanded on it. Recent research found that adult drivers with ADHD are more prone to road rage and more likely to use their vehicles aggressively.[27] A 2005 study demonstrated findings that complicate the problem: Drivers with ADHD tend to overestimate their driving skills relative to their actual driving ability, not recognizing that they have a problem despite higher incidences of crashes, speeding citations, and suspended or revoked licenses.[28]

Compared to age-matched peer control groups, research shows that adults with ADHD are:[1,21-23,25,29,30]

> ► Two to four times more likely to have been in a car crash

> ► Two to four times more likely to have been in multiple crashes throughout driving histories

> ► Involved in significantly worse car crashes, as indexed by the dollar amount of damage and the likelihood of bodily injuries

> ► Two to three times more likely to receive speeding citations

> ► Two to four times more likely to have their driver's licenses suspended or revoked

The Milwaukee study found that persistent ADHD (the H+ group) was associated with more driving problems than was childhood ADHD that did not persist into the adult years (the H- group).

Research shows that these driving risks apparently are not the consequence of the disorders commonly comorbid with ADHD, such as oppositional and conduct disorder, anxiety, or depression. Instead, they seem to stem directly from ADHD.[31] More recent research has shown that alcohol may significantly impair driving abilities of adults with ADHD, even more than it impairs driving abilities of those without ADHD.[32] Just as importantly, research has shown that ADHD medications, particularly stimulants, appear to improve the driving performance of teens and adults with ADHD.[33] Whether this benefit also reduces their risk of driving problems such as citations or crashes is unknown, as no studies have persisted long enough to measure such an effect.

One study suggested that teens with ADHD drive a manual transmission vehicle rather than drive an automatic because it focuses their attention on driving and provides them with more greatly stimulating activity while driving.[34]

These and other findings show that ADHD in adults has the potential to adversely affect every major life activity studied to date, more than most other outpatient psychiatric disorders.

How Does ADHD Change Its Presentation Across the Lifespan?

Although the major symptom constructs involved in ADHD remain the same from childhood to adulthood (inattention, poor inhibition, and generally reduced self-regulation), the symptoms of each construct may appear differently at different periods in a patient's life (see Table 1.2).

Table 1.2   Characteristics of ADHD Across the Lifespan[2,5,14,19,21,31,35,36,37]

Symptom	Childhood	Adolescence	Adulthood
Inattention	• Making careless mistakes • Being easily distracted • Failing to listen to instructions • Failing to complete school and home tasks • Disorganization • Forgetfulness	• Being easily distracted • Difficulty concentrating • Failing to complete homework on time • Difficulty working independently • Poor follow-through on commitments • Becoming bored easily • Disorganization • Forgetfulness	• Failing to listen to instructions • Not completing paperwork • Feeling overwhelmed by large projects • Missing deadlines • Disorganization, especially related to time management • Forgetting commitments • Being late for appointments
Impulsivity	• Interrupting others • Blurting out answers • Not waiting one's turn	• Substance experimentation or abuse • Unprotected sex • More sexual partners • Temper outbursts • Driving too fast • Car crashes • Interrupting others	• Excessive use of alcohol and tobacco • Substance experimentation or abuse • Driving too fast • Car crashes • Temper outbursts • Impulsive job changes • Interrupting others • Impulsive spending • Extramarital or cohabiting affairs
Hyperactivity	• Fidgeting and squirming • Inappropriately running or jumping • Inability to play or perform activities quietly • Highly overactive behavior, as if "driven by a motor"	• Feeling "restless" and "edgy" • Appearing busy but getting little done	• Restlessness • Fidgeting • Talking excessively • Self-selecting more active jobs

Outward hyperactive behavior may arise early in childhood but diminish by adolescence and especially by adulthood. On the other hand, inattentive symptoms arise somewhat later in life but are more persistent and may even become more pronounced in adulthood. Adults with ADHD, therefore, are likely to have greater problems with attention, persistence, distractibility, and self-control. Patients may not be obviously hyperactive, but may report a more subjective or internal sense of restlessness, may talk excessively, and may feel a need to be busy doing things.[1,2]

Adults with ADHD tend to experience increased cognitive impairments, best described as deficits in *executive functioning*. These deficits include:[1,36,38]

- ▶ Disorganization, particularly related to time management
- ▶ Forgetfulness, especially for tasks that need to be done
- ▶ Failing to plan ahead or to anticipate future consequences
- ▶ Depending on others for maintaining order and goal-direction
- ▶ Inability to keep track of several things at once and see them to completion
- ▶ Misjudging available time and poorly managing time
- ▶ Impulsive decision-making
- ▶ Problems keeping promises and commitments to others
- ▶ Inability to stop an ongoing and often enjoyable activity to shift to a more important and urgent task

These symptoms may occur in any number of psychiatric disorders, but they are more likely to occur in adults with ADHD than with other disorders and more likely to occur in adults with ADHD than in the general population. In those with ADHD, they are especially likely to occur in combination with one another.

Executive functions are key in self-control — a person's ability to direct actions at oneself in order to change or restrain one's own behavior — thereby improving future consequences; in other words, self-regulation aimed toward the future. Self-control appears to result from proficiency in at least five major executive abilities:[36]

- ▶ Inhibition
- ▶ *Nonverbal working memory*, especially visual imagery
- ▶ *Verbal working memory*, particularly mental self-speech
- ▶ Emotional-motivational self-regulation (moderating and activating emotions)
- ▶ Planning and problem-solving (typically mental simulation)

For example, in situations that call for sitting quietly, the adult patient may experience internal restlessness or discomfort instead of displaying the overt behavior of the child who keeps climbing on things or jumping up from his seat in the classroom. The adult patient may also talk excessively rather than move about excessively in such settings.

Current models focus on deficits in executive functioning as a key element of ADHD.

executive functioning — brain functions that allow a person to plan, organize, and carry out goal-oriented behaviors

nonverbal working memory — the short-term ability to recall and process images and other nonverbal information

verbal working memory — the short-term ability to recall and process words

Many studies have found deficits in these and other executive activities in children with ADHD. Recent large studies of adults with ADHD have found many of the same deficits.[1]

What Causes ADHD?

Researchers have identified several likely causes of ADHD, with genetics being the most important and the cause of the largest number of cases. Environmental factors that may lead to impaired neurological development and functioning, starting in the prenatal period, are also responsible for ADHD, though to a lesser degree.[39]

Genetics

Almost 40 years ago, investigators noted that hyperactive (ADHD) children had more relatives with the same or related disorders. Since then, family aggregation and twin studies have confirmed a strong hereditary component to ADHD.[40] As many as 92% of monozygotic twins of patients with an ADHD diagnosis also have the disorder. Among non-twin siblings of children with ADHD, 25%–30% are also affected.[39] Adults with ADHD are far more likely to have children with the disorder—as many as 40%–54% exhibit the disorder or significant symptoms of it.[41] Numerous large studies comparing monozygotic twins with dizygotic twins have calculated that the average degree of genetic contribution to variation in the traits of ADHD is 78%. Other studies estimate that it is as high as 90%–94%.[39]

Other Factors

Other factors, including environmental biohazards that affect brain development and functioning, may contribute to ADHD. These include maternal smoking during pregnancy, prenatal exposure to alcohol and other *teratogens*, prematurity with low birth weight (especially when minor brain hemorrhaging is involved), and exposure to high levels of lead during the first few years of life. Trauma to the brain from perinatal events or head injuries is another risk factor for developing ADHD, as are brain infections, tumors, and strokes affecting the *frontal lobes*, the *basal ganglia*, or both.[39]

teratogens — substances (including medications) that cause fetal abnormalities

frontal lobe — the most anterior portion of the cerebral cortex; involved in reasoning, planning, movement, emotions, and problem-solving

basal ganglia — a group of nuclei deep within the cerebral hemispheres; involved in generation of goal-directed movement

(continues)

The Neurobiology of ADHD

Several noteworthy differences exist between the brains of people with ADHD and healthy controls. A 2002 study found significant differences in total volumes of the *cerebrum* (-3.2%) and *cerebellum* (-3.5%) in children and adolescents with ADHD compared with brain volumes in matched controls. The study showed that these abnormalities (except the *caudate* volume) persisted with age and were not the result of taking stimulant medication for the disorder, as some critics have previously claimed.[42] Other studies also found reduced functioning in the *anterior cingulate* with this disorder, in which the *dorsal anterior cingulate* fails to activate in patients with ADHD.[42,43]

As evidenced by observed symptoms, ADHD deficits most likely result from abnormalities in the *prefrontal cortex* (prefrontal lobe). The prefrontal cortex is largely responsible for the executive functions noted earlier, including verbal and nonverbal working memory, planning, impulse-control, and sustained attentiveness.[36] The 2002 study mentioned earlier, among others, also found that volumes of the frontal and temporal *gray matter*, caudate, and cerebellum correlate with ADHD severity.[44]

Experts have long theorized that imbalances in two *neurotransmitters*, specifically *dopamine* and *norepinephrine*, are the underlying causes of ADHD, noting that dopamine improves attention and decreases hyperactivity, while norepinephrine improves executive functioning and may also control impulsivity. Strong evidence supports the role of these neurotransmitters in the development of ADHD:[39]

- ▶ Numerous studies document the efficacy of stimulant medications and atomoxetine (a *selective norepinephrine reuptake inhibitor*) in treating ADHD
- ▶ High concentrations of these neurotransmitters are in the brain regions implicated in ADHD
- ▶ Genes associated with high risk for ADHD appear to regulate these two neurotransmitters

Conclusion

The findings covered in this chapter clarify that ADHD in adults is not a fiction, myth, social construction, or mere reaction to modern hectic lifestyles or a multimedia environment. Nor is ADHD merely a trivial disorder, asset, or gift to the affected patient, as some have claimed. No study, among several hundred on ADHD in adults, has found the disorder to convey any particularly positive traits, advantages, gifts, talents, or special features beyond those seen in control groups. In contrast, all evidence shows that ADHD in adults is a serious mental disorder associated with significant life impairments.

Neuroimaging of the brains of children and adults with ADHD shows a smaller, thinner prefrontal lobe area.

(continued)

cerebrum — the largest part of the brain, consisting of the two cerebral hemispheres; associated with higher cognitive functioning such as thinking, language, and action

cerebellum — part of the brain controlling balance, motion, and coordination

caudate nucleus (caudate) — part of the brain involved in learning

anterior cingulate — part of the brain involved in autonomic nervous system functions such as blood pressure regulation, as well as in executive functions such as decision-making

dorsal anterior cingulate — part of the brain involved in rational cognition

prefrontal cortex — also known as the prefrontal lobe; primarily responsible for executive functions

gray matter — part of the brain composed of unmyelinated neurons, with a gray-brown color from capillaries and neuronal cell bodies, that forms most of the cortex and nuclei of the brain, the columns of the spinal cord, and the bodies of ganglia

neurotransmitter — a chemical messenger that enables signal communication between neurons

(continues)

(continued)

dopamine — a major neurotransmitter involved in movement and balance; also significantly involved in emotional pathways

norepinephrine — a neurotransmitter or hormone involved in fight-or-flight responses, alertness, impulsivity, and concentration

selective norepinephrine reuptake inhibitor (SNRI) — a drug that inhibits the reabsorption (reuptake) or norepinephrine by neurons, thereby increasing its availability to norepinephrine receptors

Key Concepts for Chapter One:

1. Research into adult ADHD is still evolving, but we now know that it is a legitimate and persistent adult psychiatric disorder. ADHD in adults is clearly the counterpart of the well-validated childhood disorder.

2. ADHD interferes with many major life activities such as educational and employment achievements, social relationships, sexual behavior, dating, marital or cohabiting relationships, health, money management, and driving. It may also cause problems in child-rearing.

3. ADHD has a strong genetic component, making it among the most genetically influenced of all psychiatric disorders. Nevertheless, approximately 25%–35% of all cases may arise from pre- and postnatal events that compromise brain development and function.

4. Structural and functional differences exist in the brains of children and adults with ADHD. They include reduced cerebral and cerebellar volumes and a failure of the dorsal anterior cingulate to activate in patients with ADHD.

5. The underlying cause of ADHD, while still unknown, is thought to be a result of dopamine and norepinephrine imbalances in the brain. Strong evidence, including the efficacy of stimulants and atomoxetine treatments, supports this theory.

Chapter Two:
Diagnosis and Assessment

This chapter answers the following:

▶ **What Current Diagnostic Criteria Exist for ADHD?** — This section discusses the *DSM-IV-TR* criteria for ADHD, which were developed for children only.

▶ **How May Clinicians Best Use the *DSM-IV-TR* Diagnostic Criteria When Working with Adults?** — This section provides guidelines for clinicians on how to adapt the *DSM-IV-TR* criteria for use in working with adults.

▶ **What Problems Exist in Using the *DSM-IV-TR* Criteria with Adult Patients?** — This section describes the problems inherent in using the current diagnostic criteria with adult patients with ADHD; it includes applying the *DSM-IV-TR* symptom list to adults and discusses problems with the age-of-onset criterion.

▶ **Are There Better Criteria for Diagnosing Adult ADHD Than the Current *DSM-IV-TR* Criteria?** — This section proposes a set of criteria for adult ADHD that is based on recent research and discusses differential diagnosis and comorbidity issues.

▶ **What Assessment Tools Help Diagnose Adult ADHD?** — This section describes various interviews, rating scales, and neuropsychological tests that can help with the diagnosis of ADHD in adults and discusses these tools' strengths and limitations.

S TUDIES of adult ADHD are fairly new phenomena, as is recognition of the disorder itself. For these reasons, clinicians have limited resources at their disposal when it comes to diagnosing adult ADHD and differentiating it from other psychiatric disorders with similar symptoms. This chapter discusses the currently available tools for diagnosing adult ADHD and the difficulties inherent in diagnosis. A more accurate set of diagnostic criteria that is based on recent research is proposed.

What Current Diagnostic Criteria Exist for ADHD?

The current, standard diagnostic criteria for ADHD are specified in the *Diagnostic and Statistical Manual of Mental Disorders, Fourth Edition, Text Revision (DSM-IV-TR)*.[2] These criteria list 18 symptoms in two symptom dimensions: inattention and hyperactivity-impulsivity (see Table 2.1). These symptoms are based on the childhood form of the disorder and are validated only for children.

DSM-IV-TR — Diagnostic and Statistical Manual of Mental Disorders, Fourth Edition, Text Revision; the standard text by the American Psychiatric Association that sets out the criteria for diagnosing mental disorders

Table 2.1   *DSM-IV-TR* Criteria for Diagnosing ADHD

Diagnostic Criteria for Attention-Deficit/Hyperactivity Disorder

A.   Either (1) or (2):
  (1) six (or more) of the following symptoms of **inattention** have persisted for at least 6 months to a degree that is maladaptive and inconsistent with developmental level:

  Inattention
  (a) often fails to give close attention to details or makes careless mistakes in schoolwork, work, or other activities
  (b) often has difficulty sustaining attention in tasks or play activities
  (c) often does not seem to listen when spoken to directly
  (d) often does not follow through on instructions and fails to finish schoolwork, chores, or duties in the workplace (not due to oppositional behavior or failure to understand instructions)
  (e) often has difficulty organizing tasks and activities
  (f) often avoids, dislikes, or is reluctant to engage in tasks that require sustained mental effort (such as schoolwork or homework)
  (g) often loses things necessary for tasks or activities (e.g., toys, school assignments, pencils, books, or tools)
  (h) is often easily distracted by extraneous stimuli
  (i) is often forgetful in daily activities

  (2) six (or more) of the following symptoms of **hyperactivity-impulsivity** have persisted for at least 6 months to a degree that is maladaptive and inconsistent with developmental level:

  Hyperactivity
  (a) often fidgets with hands or feet or squirms in seat
  (b) often leaves seat in classroom or in other situations in which remaining seated is expected
  (c) often runs about or climbs excessively in situations in which it is inappropriate (in adolescents or adults, may be limited to subjective feelings of restlessness)
  (d) often has difficulty playing or engaging in leisure activities quietly
  (e) is often "on the go" or often acts as if "driven by a motor"
  (f) often talks excessively

  Impulsivity
  (g) often blurts out answers before questions have been completed
  (h) often has difficulty awaiting turn
  (i) often interrupts or intrudes on others (e.g., butts into conversations or games)

B.   Some hyperactive-impulsive or inattentive symptoms that caused impairment were present before age 7 years.

C.   Some impairment from the symptoms is present in two or more settings (e.g., at school [or work] and at home).

D.   There must be clear evidence of clinically significant impairment in social, academic, or occupational functioning.

E.   The symptoms do not occur exclusively during the course of a Pervasive Developmental Disorder, Schizophrenia, or other Psychotic Disorder and are not better accounted for by another mental disorder (e.g., Mood Disorder, Anxiety Disorder, Dissociative Disorder, or a Personality Disorder).

The diagnostic codes are as follows:
  314.01 Attention-Deficit/Hyperactivity Disorder, Combined Type: if both Criteria A1 and A2 are met for the past 6 months
  314.00 Attention-Deficit/Hyperactivity Disorder, Predominantly Inattentive Type: if Criterion A1 is met but Criterion A2 is not met for the past 6 months
  314.01 Attention-Deficit/Hyperactivity Disorder, Predominantly Hyperactive–Impulsive Type: if Criterion A2 is met but Criterion A1 is not met for the past 6 months

Coding note: For individuals (especially adolescents and adults) who currently have symptoms that no longer meet full criteria, "In Partial Remission" should be specified.

Note. Adapted from *Diagnostic and Statistical Manual of Mental Disorders, Fourth Edition, Text Revision* (pp. 92–93), by American Psychiatric Association, 2000, Washington, DC: American Psychiatric Association. Copyright 2000 by American Psychiatric Association. Adapted with permission.

How May Clinicians Best Use the *DSM-IV-TR* Diagnostic Criteria When Working with Adults?

Clinicians should become familiar with the *DSM-IV-TR* criteria, keeping in mind the manner in which the symptoms tend to present in adults versus children. A useful mnemonic for recognizing ADHD in adults is S.C.R.I.P.T. Clinicians should be alert to the possibility of ADHD in adults who exhibit problems with:

▶ **S**elf-Control

▶ **R**esponsibilities and restlessness

▶ **I**mpulse-control

▶ **P**ersistence toward tasks and goals

▶ **T**ime management and organization

In addition, an ADHD evaluation should be considered for people who experience repeated failure in self-care programs such as weight loss, smoking cessation, or substance abuse treatment.[14] Other red flags that should alert clinicians to the possibility of ADHD include:[13]

▶ A history of poor educational achievement, including failure to meet educational goals

▶ Poor occupational functioning or frequent changes in employment

▶ Workers' compensation claims

▶ Poor driving performance

▶ Accidental injuries secondary to risk-taking

▶ Poor satisfaction with interpersonal relationships

▶ Chronic credit or money management problems

▶ Teen pregnancy and sexually transmitted diseases

▶ Substance dependence and abuse disorders

▶ Trouble organizing a household or raising children

▶ Poor emotional self-control

▶ Depression

ADHD can complicate and compromise treatment of several other disorders, making diagnosis and treatment of ADHD important for the proper treatment of the comorbid disorder. It is recommended that adults with the following conditions be routinely screened for ADHD, as clinicians may not readily identify ADHD in patients with other disorders. Table 2.2 outlines common psychiatric disorders and their comorbidities with ADHD.[1,8,12,23,45,46]

Table 2.2   Prevalence Rates of ADHD Comorbidity with Other Disorders[1,8,12,23,45,46]

Disorder	Prevalence Rates of Comorbid ADHD (%)
Major depressive disorder or dysthymia	27–32
Substance abuse disorders	20–30
Bipolar disorder (adult onset)	10–20
Bipolar disorder (childhood onset)	80–97
Generalized anxiety disorder	11–45

What Problems Exist in Using the *DSM-IV-TR* Criteria with Adult Patients?

With the growing recognition of adult ADHD, clinicians must extend the existing diagnostic criteria to the adult population. However, several problems arise when applying the *DSM-IV-TR* criteria to adults with ADHD.

Criteria Causing Concern in Adult ADHD Diagnosis

Clinicians should consider the following concerns and limitations when assessing adult patients, while understanding that the current criteria are still useful in diagnosing adult ADHD.[1]

Age of Onset

One of the more controversial parts in the *DSM-IV-TR* criteria is the age-of-onset restriction of 7 years (Criterion B). Even for diagnosing cases in children, this criterion has proven problematic. The *DSM-IV* field trials (all done on children) concluded that limiting the age of first symptoms to below 7 years reduced the accuracy of identification of current ADHD cases and reduced agreement with clinicians' judgments.[47] Using this criterion could exclude up to 35% of cases of some subtypes of ADHD, even though such cases meet all other criteria for the disorder.[1]

For adults, the age-7 criterion poses a sensitivity problem. A recent study found that using this age-of-onset criterion excluded nearly 50% of adults who met all other *DSM-IV* diagnostic criteria for ADHD. The study also found no differences in severity of disorder, comorbidity, or life impairments between cases that met this criterion and those that did not.[1] Other investigators have found the same result.[8]

In addition, the age stipulation poses a recall problem. In the Milwaukee study, both adults with ADHD and their parents recalled an age of onset that differed by as much as 4 years from the documented age of onset. This suggests that recall of age of onset of symptoms is not reliable enough to require it as part of formal diagnostic criteria. The study also proposed age 16 as a more appropriate threshold age for onset.[1]

When applying the current diagnostic criteria to adults, clinicians should determine whether:

▶ Credible evidence exists that the patient experienced ADHD-like symptoms in early childhood, and

▶ By the middle school years (or age 16), these symptoms led to substantial and chronic impairment across settings

The best way to determine the above is to use a combination of patient self-reported history (interview and self-report scales describing childhood symptoms), the reports of others (such as parents) who knew the patient as a child, and school records, when available.

Appropriateness of the Symptom List to Adults

Another problem with the *DSM-IV-TR* diagnostic criteria is the lack of adult relevancy of most of the symptoms and impairments listed within the diagnostic criteria. Some of these specific items, such as "climbs excessively," are irrelevant to adulthood, while others could simply be better phrased for adult contexts. While the *DSM-IV-TR* mentions work activities as a legitimate domain of impairment, it fails to consider the many other domains in which adults (as opposed to children) must function effectively and which ADHD is likely to impair. Clinicians assessing adults for ADHD should evaluate the following domains for impairment:[1]

▶ Sexual behavior
▶ Cohabiting or marital relationships
▶ Parenting
▶ Driving
▶ Money management
▶ Health maintenance
▶ Employment and career-advancement
▶ Educational achievement

Threshold for Diagnosis

The current *DSM-IV-TR* criteria require that an individual have six or more symptoms from either the inattention or hyperactivity-impulsivity symptom lists. The UMass study showed that the threshold for diagnosis in the *DSM-IV-TR* ADHD criteria is overly strict in the adult population. In fact, four or more symptoms endorsed on either the inattention or hyperactivity lists, or seven or more symptoms endorsed from both lists, correctly identified ADHD in more than 93% of referred adults and ruled out 100% of adults without ADHD.[1] Other studies yielded similar results.[48]

Presentation of ADHD in Adults

When determining the diagnosis for adult patients, clinicians should focus not only on inattention, but also on the broader domains of cognitive functioning that ADHD affects, including executive functioning, poor inhibition, and generally poor self-regulation (see pages 11–12 for a description).

The current *DSM-IV-TR* criteria do not accurately reflect what we now know about ADHD, particularly in adults. Experts now view ADHD primarily as a disorder of inhibition and executive functioning.[36,49] For example, the inattention found in the disorder appears to be related to impairments in executive functioning, especially in working memory. The *DSM-IV-TR* criteria overemphasize hyperactivity and underemphasize poor inhibition and self-regulation. This is especially problematic for adult diagnosis because maturity results in a significant reduction in hyperactive symptoms to the extent where, as found in the UMass study, such symptoms no longer have significant diagnostic utility.

Degree of Impairment

Americans with Disability Act (ADA) — Federal law providing protection against discrimination to people with disabilities; the law seeks to ensure nondiscrimination in employment and to provide people with disabilities equal access to public places, programs, and services.

Another significant problem with the *DSM-IV-TR* criteria is the lack of clear definition of impairment, leaving clinicians to define their own reference group against which to judge impairment. The definition of impairment used in the *Americans with Disability Act (ADA)* may provide some guidance.[50] Under the ADA, impairment is measured relative to an average person. To be impaired in a major life activity, the individual must function significantly below the norm (the average for a person of similar background).

Two other standards for determining impairment are often used in academic settings:

▶ The intra-person discrepancy standard, in which IQ typically serves as the benchmark against which other abilities are compared and judged to be signs of impairment, if significantly discrepant.

▶ The specialized peer-group standard, in which the immediate and comparable (though highly specialized, educated, or competent) peer group is judged as the standard (as it is in colleges, graduate schools, and professions) against which a person's performance is judged. If found to be substantially different, the performance is concluded to be an impairment.

Both of these methods have substantial problems that are sufficient to rule them out as a general basis for judging impairment, in general because they fail to adequately identify impairment relative to the average person.

Challenges of Diagnosing ADHD in Adults

Clinicians face several challenges that make the accurate diagnosis of adult ADHD difficult, including the lack of symptoms specific to ADHD, lack of objective quantitative measures, *malingering*, and under-reporting of symptoms.

Lack of Specificity

Inattention in particular is a nonspecific symptom found in virtually all psychiatric disorders. Among the various types of inattention documented in neuropsychology (i.e., alertness, arousal, focused attention, divided attention, etc.), ADHD chiefly affects the capacity for sustained persistence toward goals, resistance to distraction during such persistence, and task reengagement following task disruption (which is thought to involve working memory). While impulsivity is more specific to ADHD, it is also present during manic episodes in bipolar disorder. The chronicity of poor inhibition is more pertinent to ADHD, while the periodic form is more associated with manic episodes. Hyperactivity, as noted, is not a useful diagnostic symptom for adults because it declines markedly over time in those with ADHD. Correct ADHD diagnosis should rely both on the constellation of these symptoms, especially in executive functioning, that were present chronically before age 16 and on the pervasiveness of these symptoms and their consequences across several major life domains.

Lack of Objective Quantitative Measures

No mental disorders and few medical disorders have objective tests that are foolproof for reaching a diagnosis. That this is also true of ADHD does not undercut its validity as a disorder. Because ADHD symptoms are, at their core, extremes of normal human behavior patterns, determining what constitutes a symptomatic level for a behavior is somewhat subjective, especially in borderline and mild cases of the disorder. Nevertheless, it is traditional in clinical psychology to view symptom severity that rises to the 93rd percentile (+1.5 standard deviations above the normal mean) to be indicative of statistical rarity or developmental inappropriateness, and this could be used as an initial standard here. This approach should encourage the use of standardized behavior rating scales of ADHD symptoms with adults (see assessment tools on pages 30–34) in which adequate norms are available to assist with this determination. More important than an arbitrarily chosen cutoff point for age

malingering — the deliberate feigning of an illness or disability to achieve a particular desired outcome, such as financial gain or escaping responsibility

inappropriateness, such as the 93rd percentile, is the requirement that symptoms be severe enough to produce impairment
in one or more major life activities. Disorders begin where
impairment begins.

Malingering

Clinicians should examine the "paper trail" of impairment within the available archival records (school, driving, criminal, employment, etc.) for its consistency with patient reports and the history provided.

Clinicians should be alert to exaggerated reporting of symptoms.
Patients may exaggerate the severity or frequency of symptoms
to obtain disability benefits, legal settlements, or a stimulant prescription. While researchers have found in general that adults
with ADHD are reasonably reliable reporters of their symptoms
and impairments, there is some tendency to exaggerate in such
reports when an immediate, important consequence hinges on
the diagnosis. Exaggeration of symptoms to get a diagnosis is
not usually the norm among patients coming to clinics for ADHD
in adults, but 10%–20% of patients so referred may be involved
in legal or other proceedings in which there is a direct, immediate, and sometimes financial benefit for having the disorder.[1] In
such cases, clinicians must carefully evaluate, and especially
corroborate, reports through others who know the patient well,
by conducting a careful history back to childhood.

Under-Reporting of Impairment

More typical in routine practice than malingering is the tendency
of patients who received a diagnosis in childhood and were followed to adulthood to under-report the severity of their ADHD
symptoms, at least until age 27–30. Results from the Milwaukee
follow-up study found little correspondence between self- and
other (parent) reports at ages 15 and 21 (correlations of .21 or
lower), but found an increase in convergence between sources
by age 27 (correlations around .43). Studies of adults with
ADHD in their 30s or later show good concordance between
sources (correlations of .74 or greater). This underscores the
recommendation to corroborate patient reports with the reports
of others, especially for those younger than age 30. Even among
those over age 30, as found in the UMass study, there is some
tendency to under-report the extent of impairments as opposed
to symptoms.[1]

Are There Better Criteria for Diagnosing Adult ADHD Than the Current *DSM-IV-TR* Criteria?

The recent Milwaukee and UMass research studies began with a pool of 91 new symptoms generated from chart reviews listing the most common complaints of several hundred ADHD cases and items generated from current theories of the components of executive functioning. Researchers analyzed the best symptoms for accurately classifying adults with ADHD relative to both community adults and, more importantly, adults with psychiatric disorders other than ADHD. They then tested these symptoms against the 18 listed in the *DSM-IV-TR* and identified nine out of the original list of 91 that are best suited for diagnosing ADHD in adults. There is some overlap between the new list and the symptom list in the *DSM-IV-TR.*

The new symptom list focuses heavily on executive functioning impairments, which, as Chapter One explains, are the main deficits in adult ADHD. The symptoms on this list are statistically better at diagnosing adult ADHD than the *DSM-IV-TR* criteria. When these symptoms are combined with the requirement that the onset of symptoms producing impairment be sometime during childhood or adolescence (i.e., age 16 or younger), clinicians have a more useful set of criteria for recognizing adults with ADHD.[1]

The nine diagnostic symptoms most often observed in cases of adult ADHD are listed below.[1] The adult with ADHD typically:

1. Is easily distracted by extraneous stimuli (*DSM-IV-TR* Symptom 1h)
2. Makes decisions impulsively
3. Has difficulty stopping activities or behavior when they should do so
4. Starts a project or task without reading or listening to directions carefully
5. Shows poor follow-through on promises or commitments they may make to others (*DSM-IV-TR* Symptom 1d)
6. Has trouble completing tasks in their proper order
7. Is more likely to drive a motor vehicle much faster than others (engage in excessive speeding). (If the person has no driving history, substitute: "Has difficulty engaging in leisure activities or doing fun things quietly.") (*DSM-IV-TR* Symptom 2d)
8. Has difficulty paying attention to tasks and leisure activities (*DSM-IV-TR* Symptom 1b)
9. Has difficulty organizing tasks and activities (*DSM-IV-TR* Symptom 1e)

Differential Diagnosis

It can be important for clinicians to corroborate the patient's self-report with reports from other key people in the patient's life who are reasonably familiar with the patient's history, such as a spouse, sibling, parent, or cohabiting partner.

Differentiating adult ADHD from other disorders can be challenging and requires that clinicians pay attention to the core features that distinguish one disorder from another. Inattention and problems with concentration may often be a reason for referral and evaluation, but it is important to rule out other possible explanations for these symptoms. The causes listed below (and many other conditions), while resulting in inattention, are unlikely to produce the full spectrum of ADHD symptoms, especially problems with persistence toward tasks and goals, resistance to distractions, and working memory (task reengagement after interruptions). Most telling for the clinician is that none of the other conditions is known to produce poor chronic impulsivity and poor self-regulation dating back to childhood—the hallmarks of ADHD. Clinicians should focus on the presence of more than just vague complaints of inattention. They should investigate the presence of symptoms such as poor inhibition, distractibility, self-control, organization and time management, and other executive problems that would indicate that an ADHD diagnosis is appropriate.

The following items discuss factors to consider when ruling out other disorders and making an ADHD differential diagnosis:

The history of patients with ADHD will probably include teachers' complaints of hyperactivity, poor inhibition, or inattention at school.

▸ **Evaluate the onset, chronicity, and severity of the symptoms** — Nearly all disorders produce inattentiveness, and many produce other symptoms similar to ADHD, but no other disorder produces the early-onset, chronic, and impairing impulsiveness, distractibility, lack of persistence, and executive and self-regulatory deficits that ADHD causes. Especially telling is whether the inattentiveness developed after 16 years of age, in which case clinicians should look for another diagnosis, such as mood or anxiety disorders.

▸ **Examine stressful, immediate life events** — In general, adults are likely to be exposed to life stressors that can produce ADHD-like symptoms, especially if clinicians excessively focus on inattention. These include health crises, loss through death or relationship failures, and major career changes. Unlike ADHD symptoms, however, stress symptoms and resulting disorders such as depression do not create significant problems with inhibition, self-regulation and chronic impairment that go back to childhood. Moreover, the nature of inattention in these other conditions is more akin to poor focus of attention, as seen in frequent staring, daydreaming, being easily confused or "in a fog," and slowness in initiating new activities. Patients suffering stress may also experience sluggish or intermittent processing of ongoing information, most likely from being mentally preoccupied with the stressor or dysphoric mood state.

▶ **Recognize other medical or health disorders that can mimic symptoms of ADHD**—Such disorders include:

- ■ Fatigue, which can cause inattentiveness in school, college, or work

- ■ Periodic inner ear infections, allergies, and occasional colds, which may cause inattentiveness during illnesses

- ■ Side effects from medical treatments such as chemotherapy or surgery, which may cause inattentiveness or memory problems

- ■ Side effects of many medications that cause inattentiveness or drowsiness

- ■ Chronic health conditions such as diabetes, high or low blood pressure, hypothyroidism, or hyperthyroidism, which may also reduce attention

- ■ Decline of working memory in later life (especially after age 50 for men and during peri-menopause for women), which can mimic the inattentiveness and forgetfulness caused by ADHD but is not associated with poor inhibition, does not date back to childhood, and is otherwise not associated with poor self-regulation

▶ **Rule out the presence of other psychiatric disorders as a better explanation for the presenting complaints** — Bipolar disorder, panic attacks, generalized anxiety, PTSD, and many other disorders can interfere with attention and, in the case of bipolar disorder, even inhibition. Clinicians must ensure that these disorders alone do not explain the patient's presenting symptoms. Determining if the onset of inattention corresponds to the onset of these disorders can be helpful in determining whether the inattention either is secondary to another disorder or predates the development of these disorders and could reflect ADHD. Specific disorders to consider in differential diagnosis include bipolar disorder, substance use and abuse, major depression, anxiety disorders, and borderline personality disorder.

Bipolar Disorder (BPD)

Symptoms of inattention, hyperactivity, impulsivity, distractibility, and lack of emotional control are common in both BPD and ADHD. In BPD type I, the presence of delusions, frank manic episodes, excessive elation for the context, and highly grandiose thinking helps in making the differential diagnosis. BPD type I is also marked by possible psychosis and paranoia, irrational thinking, prolonged insomnia, hypersexuality, and severe mood swings between dysphoric and manic poles, none of which are typical symptoms of ADHD. However, it is harder to differentiate BPD type II from ADHD. Below are some clues that may be helpful in differentiating the two disorders:

While those with ADHD do not typically show elevated rates of bipolar disorder, individuals with BPD, especially with childhood onset, have a higher risk of comorbid ADHD (80%–97% for childhood onset BPD).[1]

Patients with bipolar disorder type I have experienced at least one true manic episode. Patients with bipolar disorder type II experience hypomanic episodes, which are similar to manic episodes but do not cause marked impairment in functioning.

- ▶ True euphoria, with a denial of any problems on the patient's part, is a sign of BPD.

- ▶ Insomnia, especially several nights of utter sleeplessness, is common in BPD but unusual in ADHD, where the problem is often one of delayed onset of sleep.

- ▶ BPD usually starts in late adolescence or young adulthood, while ADHD starts in early childhood in many cases.

- ▶ ADHD is chronic and persistent, while BPD is cyclical or episodic and characterized by bursts of behavior that are obviously abnormal for the person.

- ▶ Adults with mania or hypomania demonstrate inappropriate levels of euphoria, which is not characteristic of ADHD. In ADHD, many adults experience relatively chronic demoralization at their checkered history of failures to attain goals and less than expected achievements. BPD also requires periods of major depression, which is not a hallmark of ADHD.

- ▶ A family history of severe mood disorders, especially BPD, makes a BPD diagnosis more likely. BPD is not more common among relatives of ADHD patients but is 7–8 times more common among relatives of patients with BPD, especially those with childhood onset. Similarly, a family history of ADHD, but not BPD, makes an ADHD diagnosis more likely.[1]

Substance Use and Abuse

Inattention, memory problems, and mood swings are common traits among substance abusers. This may be due in part to the fact that 20%–30% or more of patients who abuse substances also have adult ADHD.[51] But even without comorbid presence of ADHD, many substances, if abused, can create difficulties with attention. These factors make the diagnosis of ADHD in those with drug use problems more difficult but not impossible. In some cases, substance abuse in adults with ADHD results from attempts at self-medication, especially when nicotine or other stimulants are overused. Because these drugs can have some beneficial effects on ADHD symptoms, patients may use them for self-treatment despite their harmful side effects. Preliminary research indicates that proper medication treatment for ADHD may help avoid substance abuse problems later in life.[35]

To differentiate substance abuse from ADHD, the clinician should assess if ADHD symptoms:

- ▶ Were present before the substance abuse started (indicating ADHD)
- ▶ Disappeared during periods of sobriety that lasted at least several months (indicating substance abuse disorder)

The *Michigan Alcohol Screening Test*[52] is a 27-item, validated screening scale for past and present substance use and abuse. This scale can be used during the clinical interview. A spouse, parent, or other individual familiar with the patient should also take this survey to corroborate the patient's answers.

Major Depression

Difficulty concentrating, inability to finish tasks, memory problems, and demoralization are common traits of both ADHD and major depression. However, there are distinctive differences between the two:

- ▶ In major depression, the depressed mood is more severe and may continue despite ADHD medication treatment.
- ▶ In major depression, mood states are episodic. In ADHD, down moods often reflect emotional reactions to stressful events.
- ▶ Major depression can lead to appetite abnormalities, which are typically episodic and associated with the altered mood.
- ▶ A recent history of a stressful or traumatic event, preceding and probably leading to depressive symptoms, also points to major depression rather than ADHD.

Up to 40% of patients in treatment for substance abuse disorders also have ADHD.[1,2]

Substance abuse is a frequent comorbid condition in adults with ADHD that can easily complicate ADHD management. Though clinicians should resolve active abuse before ADHD treatment begins, treating ADHD may help the patient continue with drug treatment protocols.

When patients with ADHD experience difficulties falling asleep, it often seems to be the result of engaging in over-stimulating activities at customary bedtimes (playing videogames, watching TV, partying or socializing with others, etc.) or becoming so focused on an interesting activity as to forget to go to sleep at a more typical bedtime.

self-esteem — an understanding or belief about oneself

There is considerable comorbidity between anxiety disorders and ADHD. While children with ADHD may have a 25% risk for any anxiety disorder, this figure can rise to 35%–50% among adults with ADHD.[53]

Anxiety is often accompanied by inhibition, rather than the impulsivity seen with ADHD.

▶ Sleeping difficulties, either excessive sleeping or limited sleep, usually due to preoccupation with stressful events, are not typical of ADHD.

▶ Anhedonia, a loss of pleasure in previously pleasurable activities, is a major characteristic of major depression but not of ADHD.

▶ Demoralization and loss of self-confidence or *self-esteem* often result from years of untreated ADHD, years in which the patient received constant negative messages and experienced outright failures. Such symptoms of demoralization are milder than the long bouts of sadness, anhedonia, and eating and sleeping difficulties that typify major depression.

If symptoms of depression persist despite treatment for ADHD, treatment of depression should be initiated.

Anxiety Disorders

Common symptoms of both anxiety disorders and ADHD include sleeping difficulties, restlessness, work avoidance, and even irritability. Some differentiating factors are:

▶ Impulsivity is not elevated in anxiety disorders but is common in ADHD in adults.

▶ Elevated concerns, worries, or fears over the future are not typical of those with ADHD. In fact, adults with ADHD usually concern themselves far less with impending deadlines, projects, and delayed consequences than they should.

▶ Panic episodes are not typical in adults with ADHD.

▶ Anxiety disorders cause physical symptoms not associated with ADHD, such as sweating, rapid and shallow breathing, heart palpitations, and dizziness.

Borderline Personality Disorder

Impulsivity, irritability, failed relationships, and comorbidity with substance abuse are common traits in both ADHD and borderline personality disorder. Some differentiating features are:

▶ Relationships of patients with borderline personality disorder are often volatile and emotional, characteristics that stem from a fear of abandonment. Those with ADHD suffer relationship problems because of impulsive comments, a poor sense of time, a lack of follow-through on commitments, and occasional irritability over the failure and consequences of poor attention and planning.

▶ Suicidal thoughts and especially self-mutilation are more common in those with borderline personality disorder.

Comorbidity

Comorbidity of certain psychiatric disorders seems particularly high in children and adults with ADHD. More than 80% of ADHD patients in the UMass and Milwaukee studies had at least one other disorder. More than one-third of the patients had at least three comorbid conditions. The most common comorbid conditions in adults with ADHD are shown in Table 2.3.[1,3,8,12,23,45,46]

Table 2.3 Prevalence Rates of Common Comorbid Conditions in Adults with ADHD

Comorbid Diagnosis	Prevalence Rate (%)
Oppositional defiant disorder (ODD)*	24–36
Conduct disorder (CD)[1]	17–25
Substance use/abuse[1]	
• Alcohol	32–53
• Marijuana	15–21
• Other substances	8–32
Dysthymia	19–37
Major depression	16–40
Anxiety disorders, not including obsessive-compulsive disorder (OCD)	10–55

*Predicted by the presence of CD in childhood or adolescence

However, patterns of comorbid conditions differ between adults whose cases of ADHD were diagnosed in childhood and whose disorder persists into adulthood and those who were first given a diagnosis of ADHD in adulthood. Protective factors, including higher IQ and family support, may account for some of the differences in the timing of diagnosis and the types of comorbid disorders that develop in these two groups. (See the discussion of protective factors on page 6 and the different patterns of comorbid conditions and symptoms presented in Table 2.4)

Table 2.4 Comorbid Conditions and Symptoms in Adults Receiving Their First ADHD Diagnosis as Children vs. as Adults[1]

Childhood ADHD Diagnosis	Adulthood ADHD Diagnosis
• Higher risk for antisocial behavior	• Higher risk for anxiety
• Higher risk for drug use and abuse	• Higher risk for depression
• Reduced educational attainment	
• Poorer employment history	
• Lower socioeconomic status	

An ADHD evaluation is recommended for any patient who fails to respond to treatment, as ADHD may coexist with these disorders and interfere with the patient's ability to comply initially with treatment recommendations, make or keep appointments, or persist in treatment.

This large range of comorbidity prevalence rates can be explained by the fact that there are multiple studies that show a range of risks, as reflected in Table 2.3.

What Assessment Tools Help Diagnose Adult ADHD?

The following four types of assessment tools can help clinicians evaluate a patient's symptoms, impairments, comorbid disorders, and other deficits:

> ► Structured interview tools
> ► Self-reporting scales
> ► Archival records of school performance, driving, employment, credit, and criminal activity
> ► Neuropsychological tests

The typical clinical evaluation for adult ADHD does not require formal, commercially produced, structured interviews or neuropsychological testing. Rather, accurate diagnosis can be achieved through the use of traditional history-taking and records-review, combined with use of:

> ► Rating scales
> ► Traditional clinical interviews (structured to focus on ADHD diagnostic criteria)
> ► Short intelligence and achievement skills tests (used to identify any learning disabilities)

Structured Interviews

Adult ADHD Interview[54]

This interview reviews history, domains of impairment, and other relevant areas of ADHD diagnostic criteria, as well as the most common comorbid disorders likely to be present with ADHD.

Barkley's Quick Check for Adult ADHD Diagnosis

A new, validated, 18-question interview based on information from recent research,[55] this tool identifies current and childhood ADHD symptoms, as well as areas of impairment. When used alone, it should be used mainly as a screening device to assist in making the decision to conduct a more thorough clinical evaluation for ADHD.

Structured Clinical Interview for DSM-IV (SCID)[56]

With six self-contained modules, the *SCID* covers all diagnostic criteria for Axis I disorders in *DSM-IV-TR*. It is a helpful research tool in differential diagnosis and diagnosis of comorbid conditions. However, the *SCID* is cumbersome in clinical practice and does not have an ADHD module, so most clinicians are not likely to use it.

Assessment of ADHD in adults often utilizes self-report measures more than does assessment of childhood ADHD. Observations by people in the patient's life (spouse, sibling, roommate, employer) are crucial to this assessment, as adult ADHD patients often lack insight into their own behavior.

Neuropsychological testing generally focuses on sustained attention, impulsivity, and executive functioning.

The Adult ADHD Interview is a paper version of the interview used in recent research on ADHD in adults.

When asking questions about employment, clinicians should ask what specific tasks patients enjoy and what tasks they avoid. For example, they may avoid paperwork or accounting, while starting new projects may be a favorite activity. In addition, clinicians may find it useful to ask patients to rate the amount of attention needed in their work and what type of job they would like to do if they could improve their concentration.

Self-Reporting Scales

Rating scales are used to evaluate the degree of inappropriateness of symptoms relative to a patient's age and sex. However, this evaluation reflects just one criterion of the seven or more that are needed to make a diagnosis of ADHD. Alone, a scale is a screening device leading one to refer those with elevated symptoms for more thorough examination; consequently, ratings alone are never sufficient to make a diagnosis of ADHD in adults. Still, they are very useful when combined with other measures and clinical interviews in addressing all relevant *DSM-IV-TR* diagnostic criteria for ADHD, such as onset, course, impairment, and cross-situation pervasiveness, and in ruling out other disorders as explanations.

Adult ADHD Self-Report Scale (ASRS)[57]

Developed by the World Health Organization, the *ASRS* includes 18 items corresponding to the current *DSM-IV-TR* criteria for inattention, impulsivity, and hyperactivity. A screener version of six select items is known as the *ASRS Screener.*

Adult ADHD Investigator Symptom Rating Scale (AISRS)[58]

The *AISRS* is a clinician-administered, scripted scale based on the *ADHD Rating Scale IV* (*ADHD RS-IV*).[59] The questions and prompts on the *AISRS* aim specifically at adult experiences. Various clinical studies have used this tool.[60]

Barkley's Adult ADHD Quick Screen[61]

This 13-item, validated questionnaire is based on recent research and screens symptoms to identify adults who need further evaluation for ADHD.[1] Scores indicate current ADHD symptoms and impairments in major life domains.

Brown ADD Rating Scale[62]

This scale has a self-report and a "significant other" report on the same form. It measures ADHD symptoms and various executive functioning deficits.

Conners' Adult Attention-Deficit Rating Scale (CAARS)[63]

This is a 42-item, validated scale covering six areas of functioning including *DSM-IV-TR* ADHD symptoms. It also includes key items for detecting depression and anxiety, an important feature, as Table 2.4 suggests, because depression and anxiety are the most commonly diagnosed comorbid conditions in adults receiving their first ADHD diagnoses.

The *Symptom Checklist 90—Revised*[64]

This does not assess ADHD in adults but can be useful in screening for comorbid disorders. It assesses nine areas of psychopathology:

- ▶ Somatization
- ▶ Obsessive-compulsion
- ▶ Interpersonal sensitivity
- ▶ Depression
- ▶ Anxiety
- ▶ Hostility
- ▶ Phobic Anxiety
- ▶ Paranoid Ideation
- ▶ Psychoticism

Wender Utah Rating Scale (WURS)[53]

A 61-item, validated scale for rating an adult patient's childhood symptoms, the *WURS* appears to differentiate between adults with ADHD, adults with depression, and the healthy population. However, precise symptoms from the *DSM-IV-TR* are not on the scale, so its use has declined in favor of those that specifically assess *DSM-IV-TR* symptoms. If the *WURS* is used, the *DSM-IV-TR* criteria would need to be used in addition to this scale to determine the actual presence of ADHD.

Archival Records

Of considerable assistance in the diagnosis of ADHD is the obtainment and review of archival performance records for various major life activities. These include past school records (such as school transcripts and report cards retained by parents), driving records, employment history (as reflected in W-2 statements, for instance), credit reports and history, and even official criminal records. Such records can show whether longstanding symptoms have been present and have resulted in significant impairment in major life activities.

Neuropsychological Tests

Neuropsychological tests are not appropriate for diagnosis. The positive predictive power (PPP) of these tests, while often acceptable, is countered by their unacceptably high levels of negative predictive power (or false negatives). Even their high PPP is usually established through comparison to normal control groups, so their clinical utility is not especially convincing. Somewhat more helpful are demonstrations of their capacity to distinguish among other disorders and ADHD.[1]

At best, neuropsychological tests help pinpoint the patient's cognitive strengths and weaknesses. The measures themselves cannot pinpoint the cause of weaknesses they find, nor can they assess if the weaknesses result from ADHD or some other disorder. Thus, while deficits of executive functioning on any neuropsychological test may indicate the presence of a disorder or even be consistent with a diagnosis of ADHD in an adult, low test scores in isolation are not sufficient to make the diagnosis, and normal scores are not useful in ruling out the disorder.

Behavior Rating Inventory of Executive Function (BRIEF)[65]

Available in two rating forms for children, a parent questionnaire and a teacher questionnaire, this inventory is designed to assess executive functioning in the home and school environments. It provides information on how well a patient can regulate behavior, inhibit impulses, control emotions, initiate projects, use working memory, plan and organize, organize environment and materials, and monitor work. It also has three broader indices: Behavioral Regulation, Metacognition, and a Global Executive Composite score. Further, the Working Memory and Inhibit scales accurately differentiate among ADHD subtypes. An adult version of the scale became available in 2006 and may prove to be equally as useful with adults as the original version is with children.[66]

Conners' Continuous Performance Test (CPT)[67]

The CPT consists of a 14-minute, validated, computerized test that measures response to a predetermined stimulus in the presence of other, rapidly projected stimuli. The test indicates impulsivity and inattentiveness. As a group, adults with ADHD often perform more poorly than adults without ADHD on this test, particularly on measures of response time, errors, and change in reaction time speed and consistency. The test does not reliably differentiate between adults with and without ADHD.[68] As such, it is not recommended for routine clinical or diagnostic use.

Even though current research has failed to demonstrate the value of using these measures with adult populations, clinicians can make valuable observations about behavioral style, impulse control, reactivity, and attention when administering structured cognitive tasks such as the Wechsler Adult Intelligence Scale, Fourth Edition (WAIS-IV) or the Continuous Performance Test (CPT). An audio-taped guide for using the CPT as a source of behavioral observations is available.[69]

It is much less expensive to use rating scales than to conduct a complete neuropsychological test battery that measures these same executive functions (inhibition, working memory, planning, etc.). Such scales can also sample the patient's functioning in these domains over a far longer time than can neuropsychological tests, which may rely on a sampling window of just a few hours.

Stroop Word Color Test[70]

This widely used test of inhibition and resistance to distraction assesses concentration in the presence of interfering information. The examinee looks at a list of color names printed in different colors (which do not correspond to the name). The examinee has to say the color of the ink, not the word itself. It is easier and faster to read the word. Ignoring the word and saying the color of the ink takes more concentration and requires control over interference. Both children and adults with ADHD often perform this task poorly, but its accuracy for diagnosis is unacceptable for general clinical use.[1]

Wechsler Adult Intelligence Scale,
Fourth Edition (WAIS-IV)—Digit Span Subtest[71]

This subtest assesses working verbal memory. The examinee receives increasingly longer strings of numbers and must repeat them back to the examiner (in the same order on the first test, in reverse order on the second test). The test allows comparison of scores to a normative population, sorted by age group. The same caution that applies to the *CPT* applies here—the test is not accurate enough for clinical diagnosis to recommend its routine clinical use.[1]

Key Concepts for Chapter Two:

1. The *DSM-IV-TR* criteria for diagnosing ADHD were developed for children, not adults. Using these criteria for adults causes several problems. Not all symptoms in children are relevant to adults if symptom limitations are kept in mind and other means of overcoming them are implemented. There is no clear definition of impairment, the threshold for diagnosis is too restrictive, and the age criterion is unrealistic, even for diagnosis in children.

2. A list of nine criteria for identifying ADHD in adults was developed based on the UMass and Milwaukee studies and is presented in this chapter on page 23.

3. The difficulty in diagnosing adult ADHD stems from four main factors: lack of specificity, lack of objective quantitative measures, malingering, and under-reporting of symptoms.

4. Evaluation of an adult patient for possible ADHD should include ruling out other psychiatric disorders with similar symptoms. In particular, clinicians should rule out bipolar disorder, substance use and abuse, major depression, anxiety disorders, and borderline personality disorder.

5. Several psychiatric disorders show high comorbidity rates with ADHD. These disorders are oppositional defiant disorder, conduct disorder, substance use or abuse, dysthymia, major depression, and anxiety disorders (not including obsessive-compulsive disorder).

6. Three categories of assessment tools can help diagnose adult ADHD: structured interviews, self- and other reporting scales, and archival records. None of the existing tools should be used as a stand-alone diagnostic measure of adult ADHD. Rather, assessment tools, clinical histories, and interviews of patients and significant others should be used in combination.

Chapter Three:
Pharmacological Treatment

This chapter answers the following:

- ► **What Medications Are Available to Treat ADHD?** — This section outlines the U.S. FDA-approved medications available for the treatment of ADHD in adults and details the pharmacology of these medications. It also explains that medications alone, while highly beneficial, are not usually sufficient to address all impairments or comorbid disorders.

- ► **What Special Considerations Exist for Medication Treatment in Adults with ADHD?** — This section explains what clinicians should consider when prescribing medication for adult ADHD. Examples include short- vs. long-acting medications, past and present drug use and abuse, side effects, special warnings, and contraindications.

- ► **How Is ADHD Pharmacotherapy Managed?** — This section explains treatment order (first-line and second-line medications) and the need to combine medication therapy with patient and family education and cognitive-behavioral therapy.

A T the forefront of ADHD treatment are medications, most commonly stimulants. Though there is ample information on ADHD pharmacological treatment in children, much less is known about the same in adults. As a result, only five medications are currently approved by the FDA to treat adult ADHD. Because of increasing recognition of adult ADHD, emerging research will lead to more pharmacologic options in the future. This chapter looks at available, approved treatments, investigational medications, and special considerations for pharmacotherapy in the adult ADHD population. It also discusses pharmacotherapy for comorbid conditions and the importance of combining pharmacotherapy with education and *cognitive-behavioral therapy*.

cognitive-behavioral therapy — a treatment approach that uses behavior to modify thought processes, usually to counter negative ideas and perceptions

What Medications Are Available to Treat ADHD?

Medication is a major part of adult ADHD treatment and is often the primary initial intervention after diagnostic evaluation and appropriate education of the patient and family about the disorder. This section discusses stimulant medications, the nonstimulant atomoxetine, and *off-label use* of antidepressant medications.

off-label use — the clinical use of a medication for a purpose that has not been approved by the Food and Drug Administration, but may have positive research findings for a disorder.

amphetamine — a group of medications that increase dopamine and norepinephrine availability by blockade of the corresponding retake transporter and release from the pre-synaptic neurons

methylphenidate (MPH) — a stimulant medication that increases dopamine transmission by blockade of the retake transporter, leading to increased arousal

noradrenergic attention circuit — neural pathway that uses norepinephrine to modulate levels of arousal and attention

mesostriatal pathway — dopaminergic neural pathway connecting the midbrain to the basal ganglia

dorsal lateral prefrontal area — a region of the brain located near the front and to both sides of the prefrontal cortex and which is involved in working memory and attention

nigrostriatal pathway — the connection between the substantia nigra and striatum that is one of the brain's major dopamine pathways, and as such is heavily involved in movement and attention

inhibitory effects — responses in which specific neurotransmitters bind to receptors on a neuron and thereby decrease the probability that neurotransmitters will be released by that neuron

Pharmacology of ADHD Stimulant Medications

Stimulant medications are the most frequently used medications for treating ADHD. Stimulant compounds used in ADHD treatment are in two categories, *amphetamines* and *methylphenidate (MPH)*. The mechanism of action of each of the two compounds is similar, but not identical.

Methylphenidate blocks the reuptake of dopamine and to a lesser degree, norepinephrine, thereby increasing the availability of these neurotransmitters in the synapse.

Amphetamines block reuptake of norepinephrine and dopamine as well as promoting additional release of dopamine and norepinephrine from the presynaptic neuron. This action increases synaptic dopamine and norepinephrine.

This difference in mechanisms of action may account for individual response and tolerance. However, clinicians will not be able to use these differences to predict which patient will respond to which medication because efficacy in large groups is equal.

The term "stimulant" is an historical label referring to the behavioral manifestation felt by a person without ADHD, rather than the mechanism of action of the medication, or its manifestation in those with ADHD. Methylphenidate and amphetamines are rapidly absorbed into the brain and act on nerve circuits that modulate **attention** and **reward.** Behavioral effects occur in 1 to 3 hours for immediate-release preparations.

The **attention** pathway releases the neurotransmitter norepinephrine when activated. This release stimulates norepinephrine receptors, which then activate nerve cells in the cortex of the brain; this activation results in increased attention, arousal, and concentration. Norepinephrine is then reabsorbed by the nerve cells of the *noradrenergic attention circuit*.

There are two **reward** pathways that use dopamine as a neurotransmitter. The *mesostriatal pathway* activates executive functions in the *dorsal lateral prefrontal area* of the brain, while the *nigrostriatal pathway* regulates motor behavior and reward sensitivities, which focus attention on the task at hand.

Methylphenidates and amphetamines have a dual effect on nerve circuits in the brain: They enhance the availability of norepinephrine and dopamine in the nerve synapses. The effects of these medications allow for alert, focused attention, and their *inhibitory effects* shut out unwanted stimuli or responses, further allowing the patient to pay selective attention to appropriate or desired stimuli. The combination of these two effects provides the patient with a sense of control that is well beyond a simple lowering of activity level.[72]

FDA-Approved Medications for ADHD in Adults

Most pharmacological medications for ADHD were developed for the childhood disorder. With the increased recognition that ADHD persists into adulthood, research protocols in the past 10 to 15 years have sought to demonstrate efficacy in adult ADHD.

We will review the research on the current medications approved by the FDA for adult ADHD. Some medications, although not specifically approved, may be used "off-label" for which there is supporting research and individual patients may not have responded or tolerated approved agents.

The American Academy of Child and Adolescent Psychiatry (AACAP) guidelines for the treatment of ADHD in children and adolescents designates stimulants as *first-line medications* for ADHD. After unsuccessful trials of a methylphenidate and amphetamine product, atomoxetine becomes the next choice in uncomplicated ADHD.[73]

first-line medication — The medication treatment of choice, because it has proven most efficacious and well tolerated or treatment guidelines dictate greatest efficacy

Although there are no formal guidelines for the treatment of adults, it seems prudent to follow these recommendations in adults until subsequent research demonstrates otherwise.

To date, the following five medications are FDA-approved for adult ADHD:

► An extended-release preparation of mixed amphetamine salts [MAS] (Adderall® XR)

► An extended-release preparation of dexmethylphenidate (Focalin™ XR)

► A prodrug preparation of *d*-amphetamine covalently bonded to *l*-lysine, which is converted to pharmacologically active *d*-amphetamine after ingestion (Vyvanse™)

► A prolonged-release OROS formulation of methylphenidate (Concerta®)

► The norepinephrine reuptake inhibitor atomoxetine (Strattera®)

Stimulant Medications

The study of stimulants in the pediatric ADHD population goes back some 70 years ago when Dr. Bradley first described the remarkable improvement of hyperactive children treated with Benedrine.[74] Their routine use in this population began approximately 25 years ago. Their safety, efficacy, and tolerability are well established in children. To date, however, only a few dozen studies have examined the use of stimulants in the adult ADHD population. These studies show a variable response rate ranging

The stimulants are Schedule II controlled substances. As a class, these drugs have been determined by the FDA to have a high potential for abuse. Prescriptions of this class do not allow refills, thereby requiring patients to have hardcopy prescriptions from their treating clinician.

Vital signs and ADHD medications — In the trials of all FDA-approved medications for adult ADHD, group data demonstrates nominal increases in systolic blood pressure (+2–5 mm Hg), diastolic blood pressure (+x–x mm Hg) and pulse (+3–5 pbm). Although this is reassuring, there is a range of change in which outliers exist. For this reason, it is recommended that vital signs be checked prior to starting medication and regularly thereafter. Any persistent elevations need to be addressed.

from 25%–78%.[75,76] We know today that higher doses of stimulants than previously studied yield better results.[13,75-81]

The following discussion of stimulant medications primarily focuses on the FDA-approved medications for treating adults with ADHD, although there is a brief description of controlled research with off-label medications.

Dexmethylphenidate, Extended-Release

Dexmethylphenidate has a duration of action of 12 hours in pediatric trials and is marketed under the brand name Focalin™ XR (Novartis). It is available in 5, 10, 15, and 20 mg capsules. It is currently approved for the treatment of ADHD in children, adolescents, and adults with a recommended dose for adults of 20 mg once daily in the morning.

A 5-week, randomized, double-blind, placebo-controlled, fixed-dose, parallel-group study demonstrated positive results in adults with ADHD. Two hundred twenty-one randomized patients received a placebo or 20, 30, or 40 mg per day of the extended-release preparation of dexmethylphenidate. Changes from baseline, assessed on the *DSM-IV ADHD Rating Scale*, were significantly superior to placebo in all three treatment groups. All doses produced significant reduction of symptoms compared to placebo and no single dose was found to be superior.[82]

The study design does not answer the clinician's question, "If the patient doesn't respond at a low dose, what is the likelihood that the patient will respond to a higher dose?" Clinical practice suggests titrating dose to symptom reduction and functional improvement. This study design does provide information on safety and tolerability at doses to 40 mg per day. Adverse events occurring >10% in the adult controlled trial were headache, decreased appetite, insomnia, dry mouth, nausea, feeling jittery, and anxiety.[82]

Lisdexamfetamine Dimesylate (LDX)

prodrug — a chemical that is biologically inactive until converted in the body to the active therapeutic agent

Lisdexamfetamine dimesylate is a *prodrug* stimulant and represents a new class of agents for ADHD treatment. It is marketed as Vyvanse™ (Shire). Vyvanse™ is available in 20, 30, 40, 50, 60, and 70 mg capsules for once-daily dosing. Initially approved by the FDA for use in children aged 6 to 12 years, and now FDA approved for use in adults ages 18 to 55.[83]

Vyvanse™ is a therapeutically inactive molecule in which *d*-amphetamine is covalently bonded to *l*-lysine. After oral ingestion, it is converted to pharmacologically active *d*-amphetamine and *l*-lysine, a naturally occurring amino acid.[84] The extended-duration of action characteristic of Vyvanse™ is due to the conversion of the prodrug into the pharmacologically active *d*-amphetamine in a rate-limited enzymatic process.[85]

Recent research demonstrated significant improvement in ADHD symptoms in 414 adults aged 18 to 55 who were given Vyvanse™. This double-blind, placebo-controlled, forced-dose study investigated changes in ADHD symptoms over 4 weeks, with improvement seen within 1 week of treatment with Vyvanse™. Treatment at studied doses (30, 50, and 70 mg) produced significantly better improvement in ADHD symptoms than placebo, as measured by the *DSM-IV ADHD Rating Scale*. Assessment using the Clinical Global Impressions-Improvement (CGI-I)[86-88] scale also revealed improvement ranging from 57%–61%. All doses produced significant reduction of symptoms compared to placebo and no single dose was found to be superior.[89]

Treatment effects based on dose are not commonly found in forced-dose titration studies because of the statistical methods of analyses. The forced-dose study design has been utilized in most adult ADHD trials with all the agents: Adderall XR, Focalin XR, Vyvanse™.

Methylphenidate, OROS Extended Release

This formulation of extended-release methylphenidate utilizes a unique osmotic release oral system (OROS) to deliver an imediate dose of medication followed by controlled release over 9 hours although behavioral effects in pediatrics lasts to 12 hours. It is marketed under the brand name Concerta® (McNeill Pediatrics). It is available in tablet strengths of 18, 27, 36, and 54 mg and is given in once-daily dosing. Concerta® has been FDA approved for use in children and adolescents and now is approved by the FDA for use in adult ADHD ages 18 to 65.[90]

OROS® osmotic pump technology — a method of delivering oral medication through a capsule with osmotic pressure and a laser-drilled hole, that forces a very precise extended release of the medication into the gut

Results of recent double-blind, randomized, forced-dose, placebo-controlled research demonstrated efficacy of Concerta® in adults. In the European study, 401 adults with ADHD were given Concerta® (18, 36, or 72 mg per day) or a placebo for 5 weeks. Results showed that treatment with Concerta® at all prescribed doses was associated with significantly greater improvement from baseline on the Conners' Adult ADHD Rating Scale (CAARS)[63] compared with the placebo group.[91]

In the U.S. trial, 226 adults with ADHD were enrolled in a 7-week randomized, placebo-controlled, dose-titration design. Those adults assigned to Concerta were started at 36 mg once a day and titrated once a week by 18 mg up to a maximum of 108 mg daily. If the subject achieved a 30% or better improvement on the investigator-rated Adult ADHD scale and Clinical Global improvement was "much" or "very much" improved, this dose was maintained without further dose increase. Titration occurred over 5 weeks with an additional 2 weeks at maintenance dose. The results demonstrated that Concerta was effective in improving ADHD symptoms vs. placebo. In the pooled data of both trials, the most common adverse reactions (>10%) reported in adults were dry mouth, nausea, decreased appetite, headache, and insomnia.[90]

Mixed Amphetamine Salts (MAS), Extended-Release

Mixed amphetamine salts are formulated in a double-beaded, pH-dependent, extended-release preparation marketed under

Gastrointestinal alkalinizing agents include sodium bicarbonate and antacids. Coadministration of MAS and gastrointestinal alkalinizing agents may disrupt the absorption process and alter its clinical impact.

Atomoxetine is metabolized by cytochrome P450 2D6 (CYP2D6). Some people who are slow metabolizers of CYP2D6 experience increased side effects when taking this medication. In patients with normal CYP2D6 metabolism, atomoxetine dose adjustment may be required when CYP2D6 inhibitors, such as fluoxetine, paroxetine, or bupropion are coadministered.[92]

Atomoxetine, unlike the stimulant medications, does not have an immediate effect. Benefits may be noticed within the first 2 weeks for adults, while full efficacy may take 4 to 6 weeks to establish.

striatum (corpus striatum) — a part of the brain containing the caudate nucleus and involved in movement and executive functions

nucleus accumbens — part of the brain that is involved in rewards and addiction, acted upon by dopamine

(continues)

the brand name Adderall® XR (Shire). Adderall® XR is available in capsule strengths of 5, 10, 15, 20, 25, and 30 mg.

Efficacy of Adderall® XR was demonstrated in a 4-week, randomized, double-blind, forced-dose titration, placebo-controlled, parallel-group study. Two hundred fifty-five randomized patients received a placebo or 20, 40, or 60 mg per day of the extended-release preparation of MAS in one morning dose. Changes from baseline, assessed on the *DSM-IV ADHD Rating Scale*, were significantly superior to placebo in all three treatment groups. All doses produced significant reduction of symptoms compared to placebo and no single dose was found to be superior.[92] The most common adverse events reported in adults included decreased appetite, difficulty falling asleep, and dry mouth.[92]

Low gastric pH can interfere with the absorption of MAS. Conversely, alkalinizing agents, both gastric and urinary, can increase blood levels of amphetamines. Patients taking MAS should not take alkalinizing agents.[92]

Nonstimulant Medications

Atomoxetine (Strattera®)

Atomoxetine is marketed under the brand name Strattera® (Eli Lilly and Company) and is available in capsule strengths of 10, 18, 25, 40, 60, 80, and 100 mg.[93] Atomoxetine is approved for the treatment of ADHD in children, adolescents, and adults.

Atomoxetine is a nonstimulant, highly selective, norepinephrine reuptake inhibitor. The drug also increases dopamine levels indirectly in the prefrontal cortex, though not in the *striatum* or the *nucleus accumbens*. Because of its primary mechanism of action on norepinephrine, there is a delayed onset of response, approximately 2 weeks.[94] When first investigated as an antidepressant, it failed to show treatment superiority to placebos. However, inspired by successful treatments of ADHD with *tricyclic antidepressants (TCAs)*, a trial study showed that treatment with atomoxetine was superior to placebo in the pediatric ADHD population. Two identically designed, 10-week, randomized, double-blind, placebo-controlled trials with a total of 536 adults with ADHD found improvement in symptoms, measured on the *Conners' Adult ADHD Rating Scale, Screening Version (CAARS)*, were statistically significant compared with placebo.[94] Atomoxetine is generally well tolerated and has no abuse potential; the most frequently reported adverse events were dry mouth, insomnia, fatigue, and nausea.[93,94]

Postmarketing analysis yielded four reports of severe hepatotoxicity among use in more than 4 million patients who took the drug. As a result, atomoxetine now carries a bolded warning about the risk of hepatic injury. At the first sign of hepatic injury, clinicians should discontinue atomoxetine and test liver enzymes.[93] This rare hepatotoxicity appears to resemble a drug-related autoimmune response that adversely affects liver cells.

The prescribing information for Strattera® carries a black-box warning about an increased risk of suicidal thoughts in children and adolescents. According to the warning in 2005, "pooled analyses of short-term (6 to 18 weeks) placebo-controlled trials of Strattera in children and adolescents have revealed a greater risk of suicidal ideation early during treatment in those receiving Strattera, compared to placebo." There is currently no concern about a similar effect of suicidal ideation of atomoxetine on adults with ADHD. The black-box warning should be considered in light of research showing that children, teens, and adults with ADHD have significantly higher rates of suicidal thoughts and attempts than control groups. These rates peak at approximately 33% during the high school years (vs. 20%–25% for general population teens). There is also a fivefold increase in risk of suicide attempts during high school versus later in life (16% vs. 3%, respectively) in populations both with ADHD and without ADHD.[1] By age 27 in the Milwaukee study, these rates for the ADHD group had declined to 25% for suicidal thinking and 6% for attempts (vs. 12% and 3%, respectively, for controls) in the interim since leaving high school.[1]

Antidepressants

Though no antidepressants are FDA-approved for treating adult ADHD, randomized, controlled studies show that desipramine and bupropion can be effective treatments. They may also be a good choice for patients with comorbid anxiety, ongoing drug abuse issues, or comorbid depression.[95,96] Bupropion has been demonstrated to be effective for adult ADHD in 2 controlled trials and desipramine efficacy has been shown in one controlled adult trial.[95,96] For these patients, antidepressant doses for ADHD are comparable to antidepressant doses for major depression, although the ADHD response rate is less than that seen for stimulants and atomoxetine.

Dosing information of the FDA-approved medications is detailed in Table 3.1.

tricyclic antidepressants (TCAs) — a first-generation class of antidepressants. TCAs mainly inhibit reuptake of serotonin and norepinephrine, but cause significant side effects such as low blood pressure, dizziness, and weight gain.

Table 3.1   FDA-Approved Medications for Treating ADHD in Adults

Medication	Starting dose (mg/d)	Target dose (mg/d)	Maximum daily dose (mg/d)	Half-life (hours)	Duration of effect (hours)†
Atomoxetine* (Strattera®)	40	80	100	5	N/A
Dexmethylphenidate Extended-Release** (Focalin™ XR)	10.	20 or lowest effective dose	20	1.5 – 3	12
Lisdexamfetamine dimesylate (Vyvanse™)	30	30	70	1	13
Methylphenidate, (Concerta®)	18 or 36	36 or lowest effective dose	72	3.6	12
Mixed Amphetamine Salts, Extended-Release** (Adderall® XR)	20	20 or lowest effective dose	0	7 – 13	12

* Nonstimulant, not a controlled substance.

** Schedule II controlled substance.

† Duration of effect is established in pediatric trials only.

What Special Considerations Exist for Medication Treatment in Adults with ADHD?

Long- vs. Short-Acting Stimulant Medications

While stimulant medications are grouped by their duration of action in controlling symptoms throughout the day, long-acting stimulants provide more benefits not immediately obvious to patients:[97]

> ► Long-acting stimulants provide a uniform pattern of symptom relief throughout the day. Short-acting stimulants may wear off, and symptoms may worsen before the next dose (causing a *rebound effect*).

> ► Long-acting stimulants ensure better compliance because patients:
>   - Take only one dose in the morning — eliminating the need to remember multiple doses throughout the day
>   - Keep their privacy — they do not have to take their medication in public settings, such as work

The duration of action needs to be specifically defined so that the clinician can carefully titrate the dose to the longest duration and optimal reduction of symptoms. The overall benefits of

Adult ADHD patients need to provide feedback to their clinicians regarding the effects of their medications at different times during their daily schedules.

rebound effect — a temporary worsening of symptoms when the medication wears off during the day or upon abrupt discontinuation of medication

long-acting stimulants in providing symptom relief throughout the day should make them a first-choice treatment.

Medication Misuse and Abuse

Because stimulants have a potential for abuse, some clinicians prefer not to give them to patients with a history of drug abuse. However, experience shows that clinicians should not necessarily deny stimulant treatment to people who have conquered their addictions, and in general, management and treatment of the substance abuse should be initiated before treatment of the ADHD. However, if the severity of the ADHD will compromise the success of recovery, simultaneous treatment may be initiated, usually with a non-stimulant medication.

A recent study found that atomoxetine used to treat adults with ADHD and comorbid alcohol abuse reduced the number of heavy drinking days among the study participants. This study may indicate an advantage to using atomoxetine treatment in adults with ADHD who are currently struggling with alcohol dependence issues.[98]

Contraindications and Adverse Events

▶ The stimulants and atomoxetine can cause a life-threatening hypertensive crisis if given with a *monoamine oxidase inhibitor (MAOI)*, or within 14 days after the last MAOI dose.[82,92,93]

▶ Clinicians should not give stimulants or atomoxetine to patients with serious structural cardiac abnormalities, major arrhythmias, or other major cardiac problems. Stroke and sudden death cases have occurred during treatment, though it is unclear if these were treatment-related events. Clinicians should thoroughly evaluate cardiac risk factors and cardiac health before starting treatment, and they should promptly evaluate patients with treatment-emergent cardiac symptoms.[82,92,93]

▶ Stimulants and atomoxetine cause a slight increase in blood pressure and heart rate. Though these small increases in group data are not clinically significant, there were some outlying subjects who had revelant blood pressure and pulse increases. This finding suggests that clinicians should assess patients for risk factors for high blood pressure and monitor all patients with baseline vital signs and regularly during treatment with medication.[82,92,93]

▶ Stimulants can cause agitation. They are contraindicated in people with severe concurrent anxiety, agitation, or psychosis.[81]

monoamine oxidase inhibitor (MAOI) — a group of antidepressant medications that inhibit the activity of the enzyme monoamine oxidase

Treatment of Comorbid Conditions

From the psychiatric epidemiologic research, clinicians can expect that adults with ADHD will present with concurrent comorbid psychiatric conditions. Based on the largest psychiatric epidemiologic study to date, mood disorders, anxiety disorders, and substance abuse occur in 38%, 47% and 15% of adults with ADHD, respectively.[3] Therefore, treatment algorithms need to consider the presenting multiple psychiatric disorders in order to improve one disorder without worsening another.

Although the Texas Treatment Algorithm provides guidance for comorbidities in children and adolescents with ADHD, there are no formal guidelines yet established for adults.[73] However, diagnostic prioritization of comorbid disorders accompanying ADHD is helpful to formulate a pharmacologic treatment algorithm.[98]

Emerging but limited research might suggest the following prioritization of treatment:[98]

- ▶ **First**, address and manage substance and alcohol abuse
- ▶ **Second**, stabilize severe mood disorders
- ▶ **Third**, stabilize severe anxiety disorders
- ▶ **Fourth**, treat the ADHD

Studies show that treating adult ADHD in the presence of substance abuse produces a nominal improvement in ADHD symptoms and no change in the substance abuse.[99,100] So, treating ADHD in the presence of active substance abuse is not productive, because some of the cognitive deficits may be an outgrowth of the substance abuse, not the ADHD.

Although there are no controlled trials addressing the treatment of severe mood and anxiety disorders before ADHD, the medications chosen to treat ADHD have the potential of worsening untreated severe mood and anxiety disorders. So, in the absence of controlled trials, it seems prudent to treat severe mood or anxiety disorders before the ADHD. However, if the adult with ADHD has dysthymia or mild to moderate anxiety, treatment of the ADHD may ameliorate these symptoms as they could be an outgrowth of the patient's frustration and demoralization from ADHD failures.[98] Common side effects and their treatments are presented in Table 3.2.

How Is ADHD Pharmacotherapy managed?

For any treatment plan to succeed, clinicians need to outline realistic expectations and set clear goals at the start of treatment. They should educate the patient on the different treatment options so the patient can make an informed decision.

Table 3.2   Common ADHD Medication Side Effects and Their Treatments

Medication	Side Effect	Treatment*
Stimulants	Anxiety or Irritability	*Clinicians:* • Reduce dose or switch to long-acting preparation • Try different stimulant compound
	Dry Mouth	• Suck on sugarless candies, lozenges, or crushed ice to cool the mouth and give it moisture • Use a mouth rinse that enhances salivation; necessary for dental and gingival protection • Assess the contribution of concomitant medications that may worsen dry mouth
	Insomnia	• Take medication earlier in day • Omit or reduce an afternoon dose *Clinicians:* • If prescribing sustained-release formulation, consider changing to a shorter-acting formulation • Review and establish regular sleep hygiene • Consider adding clonidine or trazadone, if necessary
	Loss of Appetite	• Take medication during or after a meal • Add high caloric snacks during the day
	Nausea	• Take medication during or after a meal
	Weight Loss	• Take medication after breakfast or lunch • Try using calorie-enhancement strategies, such as drinking high-protein instant breakfasts with added ice cream
Atomoxetine	Constipation	• Drink plenty of fluids • Get adequate physical exercise • Add fiber to the diet • Consider use of laxatives or stool softeners
	Dizziness	• Avoid driving a car or operating heavy machinery if frequent dizziness is experienced • Avoid using caffeine, alcohol, and tobacco
	Dry Mouth	• Suck on sugarless candies, lozenges, or crushed ice to cool the mouth and give it moisture • Use a mouth rinse that enhances salivation; necessary for dental and gingival protection
	Insomnia	*Clinicians:* • Review and establish regular sleep hygiene • Consider adding clonidine or trazadone if necessary
	Loss of Appetite	• Take medication during or after a meal • Try eating smaller, more frequent meals
	Nausea	• Take medication during or after a meal

* Treatment items are written from the patient perspective, except where noted.

Each patient's unique circumstances, including health history and comorbid conditions, should guide the medication choice. The general treatment order is as follows:

1. First-line medications are the long-acting stimulants.[73]

   ▶ Because the stimulants produce an observable effect within 1 hour after ingestion, they are usually the initial medication of choice, except in the presence of concurrent severe anxiety, mood disorders, and substance or alcohol abuse/dependence. Atomoxetine may be a first-line choice in the active substance abuser presenting with ADHD.

   ▶ Clinicians sometimes report using a combination of atomoxetine and stimulant medications to treat ADHD. The research does not offer guidance on this combined treatment and the efficacy and safety have not been established.[101]

   ▶ Patients vary in their response and tolerance to the different stimulants. If a patient does not respond to or cannot tolerate an initial MPH medication, clinicians should switch to an amphetamine preparation, and vice versa. Patient intolerance to one preparation of MPH or amphetamine, doesn't mean they won't tolerate other preparations of the same compound.

   ▶ Clinicians should switch patients to atomoxetine if they do not respond to a trial of both MPH and amphetamine. Giving atomoxetine while tapering off stimulants appears safe at this point, although more research is needed.

2. Alternative medications are the antidepressants, i.e., bupropion and desipramine. Antidepressants are a good choice for patients with comorbid depression, as well as for those with ongoing substance abuse problems, provided the seizure risk of bupropion is considered, especially in the presence of alcohol or substance abuse.

It is best to start with one medication at a time and document response and tolerance issues before moving to an alternative agent. This will provide information over time as the clinician attempts to find the best medication for the patient. Given the high likelihood of polypharmacy, longitudinal documentation of medication combinations with response and tolerance if the only way to provide a thoughtful sequence of medication trials.

Treatment Goals

Pharmacotherapy alone is rarely sufficient in treating adult ADHD.[102] Treatment usually begins by educating the patient about the disorder: explaining the condition, available treatments, and resources to cope with the patient's significantly impaired areas of life. ADHD treatment is based on managing ongoing symptoms to reduce their impairments and prevent secondary harm to patients. Realistic treatment goals include identifying the most impaired areas in a patient's life and successfully managing the impairments; taking these steps allows the patient to function as well as possible in all major life domains.

Examples of secondary harm include educational failure, job loss or difficulties, damaged relationships, divorce, vehicle accidents and license revocations, and even injury and death.

The successful treatment of ADHD most often requires patient education, pharmacotherapy, and cognitive-behavioral therapy in combination. Cognitive-behavioral therapy is discussed in the next chapter.

Key Concepts for Chapter Three

1. Medication is a major part of ADHD treatment. The most common medications used in ADHD treatment affect dopamine and norepinephrine availability.

2. Stimulants, atomoxetine, and specific antidepressants can all treat adult ADHD.

3. The FDA has thus far approved five medications to treat adult ADHD: four long-acting stimulants and atomoxetine. Note, there are no short-acting stimulants approved by the FDA for the treatment of ADHD in adults.

4. When prescribing medication for adult ADHD, clinicians should consider factors such as how fast a medication works, what the benefits of this particular medication are, side effects, special warnings and contraindications, and a patient's medical history, comorbid psychiatric illnesses, and history of substance and/or alcohol abuse.

5. Special attention should be paid to treating ADHD in a patient with comorbid conditions. Careful identification of all coexisting psychiatric disorders is necessary in order to diagnostically prioritize these disorders that will facilitate a thoughtful pharmacological treatment sequence.

6. Medications alone are rarely enough to treat adult ADHD. Medications accompanied by psychosocial therapies tailored to the patient's needs will optimize daily functioning.

Chapter Four:
Nonpharmacological Treatment

This chapter answers the following:

▶ **What are the Goals of Psychosocial Treatment of Adult ADHD?** — This section explains how both psychoeducation and nondrug therapy may supplement medication treatment of adult ADHD with the aims of improving patients' understanding, bolstering self-esteem, and helping patients manage the effects of ADHD.

▶ **What Psychosocial Treatments Are Available for Adults with ADHD?** — This section outlines the various psychosocial treatments that are available for ADHD, including psychoeducation and cognitive-behavioral therapy.

▶ **What Unique Challenges Face Adults with ADHD? What Can Be Done to Help Adults with ADHD Cope with These Challenges?** — This section describes the challenges in multiple life domains that adults with ADHD face and provides suggestions for clinicians who treat these challenges.

N o treatment — medication or non-medication — cures ADHD. Instead, treatment can make the disorder manageable and improve the patient's quality of life. Successful management of ADHD usually involves a combination of patient and family education, cognitive-behavioral therapy (CBT), and medications for ADHD and comorbid conditions, as the National Institute of Mental Health's landmark Multimodal Treatment of ADHD (MTA) study showed.[102]

What Are the Goals of Psychosocial Treatment of Adult ADHD?

Because adult ADHD is a fairly new area of study, recommendations for nonpharmacological treatments are based mostly on anecdotes and common sense, as well as on extrapolations from efficacy studies in children. Very few randomized, controlled studies examined the efficacy and effectiveness of psychological therapy in adult ADHD; this is in contrast to the numerous studies done with children.

Nonpharmacological treatment of adult ADHD aims to educate patients and help them with emotional problems that often impair adults with ADHD. It tries to improve individuals' self-esteem and help them cope with their impairments. Ideally, it frees them from the vicious cycle of failure in many areas of life, which results in blame, anxiety, poor performance, avoidance, and substance abuse.

The MTA study was a hallmark research project that examined pharmacological and psychosocial treatment of ADHD. The study concluded that multimodal therapy — medication and psychosocial treatment — provided the best outcomes.[102]

Adults who have lived with undiagnosed ADHD since childhood may have a range of emotional problems that are as important to solve as the cognitive and neurophysiological problems. Many adults with ADHD suffer low self-esteem and demoralization after years of blame for their poor behavior or achievement. They may present with marital problems, employment difficulties, increased vague somatic complaints, or substance abuse issues. Adults with a long history of undiagnosed ADHD may also suffer from anxiety and mood disorders. Patients who experienced repetitive failures in educational, self-improvement, health maintenance, or substance use programs may choose to avoid certain tasks for fear of more failure.

Some patients are unable to tolerate stimulants for various reasons including side effects such as anxiety or insomnia.

Clinicians consider potentially 20%–50% of adults with ADHD to be nonresponders to pharmacotherapy. Even among patients who are helped by medication, core symptom reduction is less than 50% on average, although results vary widely across individuals.[103,104] Nonpharmacological therapy can help reduce, compensate for, or alleviate many previously untreated problems and prevent others from escalating and further compromising the patient's quality of life. Therapy aims to:

- ▶ Educate the patient and family about ADHD and its effects on the patient's (and family's) life
- ▶ Improve self-esteem
- ▶ Counter negative "self-talk" and manage avoidance response
- ▶ Address and manage executive functioning deficits, such as poor working memory and time management
- ▶ Provide coping strategies and behavioral techniques to improve functioning across the major life domains affected by the disorder

What Psychosocial Treatments Are Available for Adults with ADHD?

Psychosocial treatments available for adults with ADHD include psychoeducation, cognitive-behavioral therapy, and other modes of treatment, including group and couples therapy.

Psychoeducation

Psychoeducation is a key component of all psychosocial therapies. It involves teaching the patient and family about the disorder, its symptoms, its typical course, and its treatment. The patient's understanding of ADHD and its implications is an essential first step of any treatment modality.[53,105] Many patients rated understanding the condition as the most important contributor to their own treatment successes.[26]

Educating adults with ADHD about the disorder includes:[106]

> ▶ Instilling hope, optimism, and motivation so that patients can better understand the condition and be more inclined to engage in and follow through with a multimodal treatment plan

> ▶ Helping patients view their disorder from a perspective that empowers them to believe that their lives can be different, and encourages their active and enthusiastic involvement in treatment

Understanding ADHD and its implications improves a patient's self-image. Once their cases are diagnosed, patients often experience a sense of relief when they recognize that their difficulties are due to ADHD and that they can let go of negative beliefs about themselves, such as thinking that they are lazy, stupid, or bad (which are common complaints about children and adults with undiagnosed ADHD). The patient has an identifiable condition with symptoms that make sense. For a patient, even more encouraging than putting a name to the problem is knowing that they can manage the symptoms. This gives patients hope, which is an important element in motivating them to take an active part in their own treatments. When communicating the diagnosis to patients and their families, clinicians should remember the important roles of hope and knowledge in the successful management of ADHD.

Psychoeducation is especially important at the beginning of treatment but should be continued over the course of treatment. This is important because the patient's understanding of the disorder and his or her symptoms change over time, across situations, and with treatment. Patients also need to understand that they are a potent force in their own treatments and that effort and participation in therapy will have a significant impact on the final treatment outcome. Patients experience greater benefit from therapy when they do their part by actively engaging in treatment, practicing new skills, communicating honestly about obstacles they are encountering, dealing with inevitable setbacks, taking medication consistently, and making a genuine and persistent effort at accomplishing changes in their lives.[106]

Cognitive-Behavioral Therapy (CBT)

One model of adult ADHD proposes that behavioral deficits resulting from the brain's core biological abnormalities prevent patients from compensating for their impairments.[107] This inability to compensate for deficits results in continuous symptoms and symptom exacerbation. In other words, constant failure breeds avoidance, more failure, and an unwillingness to try things that were previously overwhelming. As a result, the patient's impairments may worsen over time.

In this model, the goal of cognitive-behavioral therapy is to interrupt this vicious cycle and teach patients effective ways to compensate for impairments and to manage avoidance. CBT often starts in patients whose medication use is stable. The behavioral part of the therapy teaches coping and compensation strategies, while the cognitive part is aimed at countering negative self-talk and thoughts.

The clinician should also address comorbid conditions that affect the patient's emotional well-being.

CBT focuses on the current difficulties the patient experiences, sets goals for further treatments, and allows for monitoring of both medication efficacy and any side effects. This approach is results-oriented, rather than insightful.[108] Areas to cover include:

- ▶ Time management and organizational skills (see details below)
- ▶ Control of negative emotions and ideations
- ▶ Cognitive techniques to help the patient with impulse control
- ▶ Some form of cognitive restructuring to help the patient counter or avoid negative thoughts and self-talk
- ▶ A reframing of the past from the perspective of the new diagnosis of ADHD; this should especially reinforce understanding and hope for an improved quality of life

A key step in educating patients to manage the disorder is to teach organizational and time-management skills. The following ideas may help patients improve organization:[106]

- ▶ Practice proactive planning by setting aside time every evening to plan for the next day. Get needed materials ready (e.g., books, clothes, keys, phone numbers, medication, important papers), pack the car the night before, or do anything else that will prevent frantic chaos the next day.

- ▶ Learn how to make an effective and reasonable "to do" list of important tasks and priorities that the patient can keep close at all times. Make copies in case it gets lost or misplaced.

- ▶ Use reminders to keep important tasks visually in sight by posting appointments, "to do" lists, or schedules in strategic areas at home and at work.

- ▶ Practice using an appointment book, Palm Pilot or personal digital assistant (PDA), or a daily planning calendar and learn to write down appointments and commitments immediately.

- ▶ Keep notepads in strategic locations (car, bathroom, bedroom, etc.), or have a portable handheld recorder handy to capture important ideas and thoughts to remember.

- ▶ Learn and practice time-management skills. Purchase a programmable alarm watch to provide cues to keep track of time.

- ▶ Use a color-coded file system, desk and closet organizers, storage boxes, or other organizational devices to reduce clutter and improve efficiency and structure in the patient's life. Consider hiring a professional organizer to assist in creating a workable system, which may include ensuring bills are paid on time, the checkbook is balanced, and living space is uncluttered.

- ▶ Make multiple sets of keys, so losing them does not become a disaster.

A key to behavioral and organizational management is to ensure that each step is explicitly understood and structured, possibly even written down.

Clinicians should prepare patients for setbacks and assure them it does not mean the methods are not working. They should reframe setbacks as learning opportunities and emphasize that changing habits and acquiring new skills takes time and practice. Individual counseling sessions that also emphasize the patient's strengths should help to counter any entrenched, negative self-image.

One CBT treatment plan researched in adults with ADHD spanned 12 to 15 sessions, had homework assignments between sessions, and comprised three core modules:[107]

This study highlighted the usefulness of using the "one location" method for reminders, appointments, and task lists. They suggest that adults with ADHD should use only **one** calendar, notebook, personal digital assistant (PDA), or computer to keep track of all of these items.

1. **Organizing and planning** — The first module involved four sessions focused on psychoeducation, which included maintaining a notebook with a task list and calendar system, using problem-solving skills, learning to break down projects to small tasks, and learning to generate action plans. Patients learned a ranking system to help them distinguish easy but less important tasks from priority tasks that they should complete first.

2. **Coping with distractibility** — The second module involved three sessions that began with measuring the patient's attention span using timed assignments. Patients then learned to divide their tasks (using methods from the first module) into chunks that fit the lengths of their individual attention spans. Patients also learned techniques to delay and reduce distractions and to schedule effective breaks.

3. **Cognitive restructuring** — The final core module focused on cognitive restructuring techniques adapted from Beck.[109] Patients were taught adaptive thinking skills and learned to use these skills during times of stress. They also learned to apply them to difficulties produced by ADHD symptoms.

Participants completed optional modules if they demonstrated difficulties with procrastination, anger and frustration management, or communication skills.

The researchers found that patients receiving this CBT therapy in addition to pharmacotherapy demonstrated more improvement in ADHD symptoms and significantly reduced anxiety and depression than patients receiving pharmacotherapy alone. Benefits remained significant after controlling for depression (which is very responsive to CBT).[107]

Other Treatment Modalities for Adults with ADHD

Research has found that multimodal treatment of ADHD is the most successful.[102] The inclusion of other people in the patient's treatment, whether they are support persons, spouses, or others with the same disorder, may improve treatment outcomes.

Support Person

Australian researchers tested a treatment involving the patient and a support person.[110] The rationale for providing a support person during treatment was that the support person could act as a coach and assist the patient in maintaining focus on the treatment program. The support person was trained to:

- ▶ Remind the patient to attend sessions
- ▶ Attend and take notes during sessions
- ▶ Assist with homework between sessions
- ▶ Make at least one phone call to the patient between sessions

Treatment consisted of eight 2-hour group sessions focused on teaching strategies to improve motivation, concentration, listening, impulsivity, organization, anger management, and self-esteem. The treatment also included homework and a workbook with exercises. Though the study relied on self-reports for assessment, participants reported improved organizational skills, reduced ADHD symptoms, improved self-esteem, and reduced anger problems. They maintained these gains at a 1-year follow-up.[110]

Couples Therapy

Patients with ADHD often have marital and relationship difficulties. Symptoms may cause the spouses or partners of people with undiagnosed ADHD to see them as uncaring, irresponsible, or inconsiderate. Partners may complain that their spouses with undiagnosed ADHD do not finish household projects or that they are poor listeners, unreliable, forgetful, self-centered or insensitive, distant or preoccupied, messy, or irresponsible. Couples therapy can help patients and their partners unite instead of fight. Both partners, however, should realize that therapy can succeed only if:

- ▶ The patient is committed to changing and managing his or her symptoms
- ▶ The patient's partner does not blame the patient but rather works with him or her toward a common goal

Experts recommend that couples divide their household responsibilities somewhat differently than usual. The adult without ADHD should do the time-sensitive tasks, such as paying bills and getting kids to school and picking them up on time. The adult with ADHD can do the less time-sensitive tasks, such as house work, yard care, getting children bathed and ready for bed.

Couples are likely to achieve that common goal only if the partner without ADHD understands the neurobiological basis of ADHD and its relatively chronic nature. That understanding helps them overcome tendencies to moralize about the patient's deficits or view them simply as character flaws or choices to act irresponsibly. Couples therapy should include a clear definition of expectations and an understanding of each person's needs in the relationship. Successful couples therapy will help the couple understand the effects of ADHD on their relationship and help both people work as a team to counter the effects of the patient's impairments.

Group Therapy

Participation in a therapy or support group has several benefits:[1,106]

- ► Patients realize that they are not alone with their problems

- ► Group sessions are excellent opportunities for information exchange and education about treatments, coping, and symptom-management strategies

- ► Group sessions let patients learn new social skills in a safe environment, when the consequences of failing are not as potentially devastating as those in the "real world"

Organizations such as Children and Adults with Attention Deficit Disorder (www.chadd.org) or the Attention Deficit Disorders Association (www.add.org) are good resources for finding support groups.

Such groups can cover medication issues, organizational skills, listening/interpersonal skills, anger control, decision-making, stress reduction, vocational/workplace issues, and personal coping strategies. To maximize the benefits of group therapy, the group should be small (10 people at most), led by a skilled therapist, and have a preset structure, such as a presentation followed by a discussion and question-and-answer session.[106]

What Unique Challenges Face Adults with ADHD? What Can Be Done to Help Adults with ADHD Cope with These Challenges?

The challenges facing adults with ADHD differ from those facing children. As discussed in Chapter One, ADHD affects a broad range of life domains in adults, including health, relationships and parenting, education, employment, finances, and driving safety.[1] Strategies for coping with ADHD symptoms across these domains are discussed below.

Health

Adults with ADHD have more difficulty managing their health and health care than those without ADHD.[1] The following strategies may be useful in helping adults with ADHD manage their health:

- ► Enlist a support person (such as a spouse or therapist) to remind and encourage the patient to get annual physicals and dental checkups so they can monitor their overall health

- ► Consider substance abuse treatment and smoking cessations programs, as appropriate

- ► Get adequate and regular aerobic exercise

- ► Learn about good nutrition and how it affects both general health and ADHD symptoms

- ► Receive treatment for comorbid disorders, such as depression or anxiety

Sexual Health

Research has shown that adults with ADHD have a higher number of sexual partners and are more likely to engage in unprotected sex.[1] Therefore, adults with ADHD should receive safer sex information, guidance, and counseling on testing for HIV and other sexually transmitted diseases, when appropriate.

Relationships and Child Rearing

Couples counseling (discussed on page 57) may prove useful in helping couples cope with relationship issues.

Adults with ADHD face challenges in maintaining healthy relationships with their spouses or partners and in child rearing. Other strategies that may improve life at home for adults with ADHD include:

- ▶ Assigning manual chores to the partner with ADHD and detail-oriented household duties (e.g., money management and scheduling of appointments) to the partner without ADHD

- ▶ Rewarding and acknowledging both spouses for completing tasks and goals

- ▶ Permitting the partner without ADHD periodic time for hobbies or trips away from home

- ▶ Finding a location to get away from others to recuperate from an upset or argument

- ▶ Taking formal courses in child behavior management, especially ones that focus on managing childhood ADHD, given the large number of adults with ADHD who have children with ADHD

- ▶ Using shared parenting, where parents alternate evenings in which each is responsible for childcare and homework

- ▶ Developing a nonverbal cueing system between the partners to signal when the partner with ADHD is talking too much, being overly emotional, or being socially inappropriate

- ▶ Getting regular aerobic exercise, such as running or walking, to help control hyperactivity and subjective feelings of restlessness

- ▶ Hiring an organizational specialist to help with home and home office organization

- ▶ Showing appreciation to family members for assistance with providing structure and support

Education

Specific challenges also confront adults with ADHD who are attending college or venturing out into the job market. These challenges include managing the disorder in the context of college or vocational training.

College and Vocational Training

Young adults with ADHD must decide if the disorder interferes with formal schooling to the extent that college is not the best option for them. These patients may choose to pursue vocational training or careers that do not require a college degree.

For those who do decide to attend college, strategies that promote success in a college environment include:

Vocational training programs offer specialized instruction to help students develop the knowledge and skills necessary to perform a specific job.

- ► Choosing a college with small class sizes that allow for individualized attention and instruction
- ► Studying in a group with more organized students
- ► Scheduling the most difficult courses for earlier times of day, when attention is better
- ► When reading difficult or boring material, keeping one hand moving down the center of the page to focus attention and the other hand free for note-taking
- ► Alternating studying between interesting and uninteresting subjects to maintain attention and concentration
- ► Learning time-management skills, especially to avoid falling into a cycle of staying up late and consequently oversleeping[108]
- ► Attending all faculty extra help or review sessions; taking advantage of formal study groups and discussion sections
- ► Learning SQ4R for reading comprehension (Survey, Question, Read, Recite, Review, Reflect)
- ► Surveying material, drafting questions
- ► Reading, reciting, writing, and reviewing after each paragraph or page
- ► Identifying a mentor or coach for motivation, support, and accountability
- ► Utilizing vocational or career counseling services well before graduation
- ► Taking advantage of groups or seminars offered by the college counseling center, including those on:
  - Social skills, relationships, and friendships
  - Time management and study skills

▶ Requesting a substance-free dorm

Enlisting the support and guidance of the college's disability services can be extremely valuable to students with ADHD; this office is not merely for students with physical disabilities. The disability office should have experience with setting up accommodations for students with ADHD, according to the Americans with Disabilities Act (ADA), including:

▶ Helping students set up a reasonable course schedule, including guidance toward appropriate types of courses and determination of appropriate course loads

▶ Providing note-takers for lectures; this frees students to focus on the lecture by not having to be concerned about recording important points for future reference

▶ Securing written outlines or notes of lectures from faculty members

▶ Providing extended time for test-taking so that students can take "time off the clock"; this involves taking tests in shorter blocks of questions and then signaling when a break is desired, at which point timing on the test ceases. After a few minutes, the patient resumes testing and the timer is started again.

▶ Alerting faculty members to the student's condition, as necessary

▶ Getting formal tutoring help with courses that prove most challenging and help with time-management skills

Employment

Adults with ADHD face challenges in maintaining employment, completing tasks on the job, and managing their workloads, among other issues.[1] Personal coaching and vocational counseling can help patients manage their workloads and perform effectively on the job. Below are some general strategies for success at work.

Personal Coaching

Personal coaching involves working one-on-one with a professional coach who advises, encourages, and gives feedback. Coaches can work daily, by phone, or by email. Patients drive the process by deciding what goals they want to achieve at home, at work, or in any other major life areas. Many adults with ADHD have difficulty persisting in tasks and often are not motivated to finish them. The coach can help the person with ADHD stay on task by offering encouragement, support, structure, accountability, and, when needed, gentle confrontation.

Vocational Counseling

Vocational counseling helps patients understand their strengths and weaknesses in the workplace. It can help them find appropriate employment that lets them capitalize on these strengths and succeed despite their impairments. In general, ADHD-friendly jobs have room for flexibility of time and organization, frequent movement, more manual activities, less emphasis on long-term planning ability, and more frequent supervision. Unsuitable jobs for adults with ADHD are ones with too many timeline pressures or too little structure. In these cases, the patient is unlikely to succeed.[111]

General Strategies for Success at Work

The following are tips to help adults with ADHD succeed at work:[106,108]

▶ Find a mentor at work. It can be a supportive coworker, a more senior and receptive employee, or even a supervisor who supports work performance improvements. Review daily goals with the mentor and report progress to this person several times a day.

▶ Break projects into small tasks and provide rewards for completing each task, perhaps with brief breaks for a drink, a quick social call to someone, or just a pause in working to think of evening or weekend pleasurable activities.

▶ Work for short periods and take short breaks between work periods.

▶ Keep anything not related to the current task off the desk.

▶ Use lists and prompts to focus on goals.

▶ Answer email and return routine phone calls once a day, at the end of the day, if feasible.

▶ Work in short bursts with brief breaks in between.

▶ Tackle the most difficult tasks early in the day when mentally fresh, rather than in mid-afternoon when more fatigued.

▶ Use aerobic exercise to renew concentration (e.g., take a brief walk, walk up and down a flight of stairs, or do a few stretches).

▶ Use timers to structure work periods (e.g., plan to work for 20 minutes on one task and set the timer accordingly).

> ► Work with others who are highly structured.

> ► Take advantage of technology that can help with organization, planning, and other difficulties that people with ADHD experience.[106] Examples of helpful technology include:

>> ■ Word processors and programs such as spell-check and grammar-check, which can help with writing, spelling, and grammar

>> ■ A variety of PDAs that can help with organization, scheduling, reminders, and maintenance of to-do lists

>> ■ Software programs and online banking systems that are available to help with personal finance, on-time bill-paying, automated savings plans, and taxes

>> ■ Books on tape and voice-activated word processing programs, which can help with the reading and writing disorders that are often associated with ADHD

> ► Declare and document the disability to receive ADA accommodations, if desired.

Finances

Managing financial matters is often difficult for adults with ADHD. People with ADHD tend to spend money impulsively, have difficulty budgeting, and save little of their incomes.[1] The following strategies can help adults with ADHD manage their finances more effectively:[106,108]

> ► For those individuals who are married or in a cohabiting relationship, the partner without ADHD should handle tasks related to money management and bill-paying.

> ► Have a monthly budget that clearly outlines recurring expenses.

> ► Use direct deposit for paychecks.

> ► Use automatic withdrawals or electronic bill-paying services for recurring expenses.

> ► Have a set percentage of income automatically deducted from the paycheck for savings.

> ► Utilize the services of a financial advisor to help with financial planning, retirement savings, and monthly budgeting. A financial advisor can provide accountability and mentoring in financial matters.

Driving Safety

Safe driving is a serious concern for adults with ADHD.[1] The following list provides strategies for improving driver safety in this population.[87]

- ▶ Take medications before driving, especially in the peak accident times of mid-afternoon and late evening; stimulants have been shown to improve the driving skills of those with ADHD.[1,29,33]

- ▶ Reduce in-vehicle distractions, such as loud music or many people talking.

- ▶ Avoid use of a cell phone while driving. Cell phones should be turned off.

- ▶ On extended trips, take frequent breaks that include short periods of aerobic exercise.

- ▶ Avoid multitasking while driving.

- ▶ Avoid speeding up to get by unexpected hazards or other cars; keeping events in front of the driver helps manage them.

- ▶ Look at the road while others are talking, not at the person talking.

- ▶ Let someone else drive after drinking alcohol or if upset.

To effectively manage adult ADHD, treatment involves multiple components including psychoeducation, individual cognitive-behavioral therapy, or other psychosocial therapy and medications.

Key Concepts for Chapter Four

1. Patient education and cognitive-behavioral therapy play key roles, along with medication treatment, in helping adults cope with ADHD.

2. Nonpharmacological methods that work well include education about ADHD and its effects, cognitive restructuring to counter negative ideations, and improving impulse control and organizational abilities.

3. Other psychosocial treatments include individual and group counseling, education, support persons and groups, couples therapy, coaching, and vocational counseling.

4. The use of technology and personal coaches can help adults with ADHD conquer the practical challenges posed by the disorder. These challenges may include timely bill payments, appointment-keeping, budgeting, and organizing tasks into manageable chunks.

5. Support persons, including mentors at work, can be an invaluable resource to the person with ADHD. They can provide feedback, reminders, and when needed, gentle guidance to keep the patient on task.

6. College students with ADHD should utilize as many of the available college services as possible, including those of the disability office, to make their college careers successful.

Glossary

A

amphetamine — a group of medications that increase dopamine and norepinephrine availability by blockade of the corresponding retake transporter and release from the pre-synaptic neurons

attention deficit/hyperactivity disorder (ADHD) — a neuropsychiatric disorder that usually becomes apparent in early childhood. Its symptoms of hyperactivity, impulsivity, and/or inattention often persist across the lifespan.

Americans with Disability Act (ADA) — Federal law providing protection against discrimination to people with disabilities; the law seeks to ensure nondiscrimination in employment and to provide people with disabilities equal access to public places, programs, and services

anterior cingulate — part of the brain involved in autonomic nervous system functions such as blood pressure regulation, as well as in executive functions such as decision-making

B

basal ganglia — a group of nuclei deep within the cerebral hemispheres; involved in generation of goal-directed movement

C

caudate nucleus (caudate) — part of the brain involved in learning

cerebellum — part of the brain controlling balance, motion, and coordination

cerebrum — the largest part of the brain, consisting of the two cerebral hemispheres; associated with higher cognitive functioning such as thinking, language, and action

cognitive-behavioral therapy — a treatment approach that uses behavior to modify thought processes, usually to counter negative ideas and perceptions

comorbid disorder — a disease or condition occurring at the same time as another disease or condition, but which is unrelated to it

D

distractibility — stimuli in the environment attract attention away from the task at hand

dopamine — a major neurotransmitter involved in movement and balance; also significantly involved in emotional pathways

dorsal anterior cingulate — part of the brain involved in rational cognition

dorsal lateral prefrontal area — a region of the brain located near the front and to both sides of the prefrontal cortex and which is involved in working memory and attention

DSM-IV-TR — *Diagnostic and Statistical Manual of Mental Disorders, Fourth Edition, Text Revision;* the standard text by the American

Psychiatric Association that sets out the criteria for diagnosing mental disorders

E

executive functioning — brain functions that allow a person to plan, organize, and carry out goal-oriented behaviors

F

first-line medication — the medication treatment of choice, because it has proven most efficacious and well-tolerated or treatment guidelines dictate greatest efficacy

frontal lobe — the most anterior portion of the cerebral cortex; involved in reasoning, planning, movement, emotions, and problem-solving

G

gray matter — part of the brain composed of unmyelinated neurons, with a gray-brown color from capillaries and neuronal cell bodies, that forms most of the cortex and nuclei of the brain, the columns of the spinal cord, and the bodies of ganglia

H

hyperactivity — a state of heightened motor and emotional activity or excitability

I

impulsivity — a lack of self-control over one's actions and words; the inability to consider the consequences of actions and words before speaking or carrying out actions

inattention — the state of being distracted, or the inability to concentrate; inattention by itself may result from a variety of physical and emotional conditions, including stress

inhibitory effects — responses in which specific neurotransmitters bind to receptors on a neuron and thereby decrease the probability that neurotransmitters will be released by that neuron

M

malingering — the deliberate feigning of an illness or disability to achieve a particular desired outcome, such as financial gain or escaping responsibility

methylphenidate (MPH) — a stimulant medication that increases dopamine transmission by blockade of the retake transporter, leading to increased arousal

mesostriatal pathway — dopaminergic neural pathway connecting the midbrain to the basal ganglia

Milwaukee study — a recently completed, NIMH-funded study of children with ADHD diagnosis followed into adulthood (mean age 27), comparing adults who still met diagnostic criteria for ADHD with those who no longer met the criteria and with a community control group who never received an ADHD diagnosis

monoamine oxidase inhibitor (MAOI) — a group of antidepressant medications that inhibit the activity of the enzyme monoamine oxidase, which in turn increases the amount of serotonin, norepinephrine, and dopamine available

N

neuropsychiatric disorder — a behavioral disorder characterized by structural and functional abnormalities of the nervous system

neurotransmitter — a chemical messenger that enables signal communication between neurons

nigrostriatal pathway — the connection between the substantia nigra and striatum that is one of the brain's major dopamine pathways, and as such is heavily involved in movement and attention

nonverbal working memory — the short-term ability to recall and process images and other nonverbal information

noradrenergic attention circuit — neural pathway that uses norepinephrine to modulate levels of arousal and attention

norepinephrine — a neurotransmitter or hormone involved in fight-or-flight responses, alertness, impulsivity, and concentration

nucleus accumbens — part of the brain that is involved in rewards and addiction, acted upon by dopamine

O

off-label use — the clinical use of a medication for a purpose that has not been approved by the Food and Drug Administration

OROS® osmotic pump technology — a method of delivering oral medication through a capsule with osmotic pressure and a laser-drilled hole that forces a very precise extended release of the medication into the gut

P

prefrontal cortex — also known as the prefrontal lobe; primarily responsible for executive functions

prodrug — a chemical that is biologically inactive until converted in the body to the active therapeutic agent

R

rebound effect — a temporary worsening of symptoms when the medication wears off during the day or upon abrupt discontinuation of medication

S

selective norepinephrine reuptake inhibitor (SNRI) — a medication that inhibits the reabsorption (reuptake) or norepinephrine by neurons, thereby increasing its availability to norepinephrine receptors

self-control — ability to direct actions at oneself to change or restrain one's own behavior

self-esteem — an understanding or belief about oneself

serotonin — a neurotransmitter active in pathways involving emotions and cognition

striatum (corpus striatum) — a part of the brain containing the caudate nucleus and involved in movement and executive functions

substantia nigra — a portion of the midbrain that is responsible for dopamine production

T

teratogens — substances (including medications) that cause fetal abnormalities

tricyclic antidepressants (TCAs) — A first-generation class of antidepressants. TCAs mainly inhibit reuptake of serotonin and norepinephrine, but cause significant side effects such as low blood pressure, dizziness, and weight gain

U

UMass study — A recently completed, NIMH-funded study comparing (1) adults not diagnosed with ADHD who self-referred to an ADHD clinic with (2) a community control group and (3) a group of patients in the same clinic who had other psychiatric disorders

V

verbal working memory — the short-term ability to recall and process words

References

1. Barkley, R.A., Murphy, K.R., and Fischer M. (2008). *ADHD in Adults: What the Science Tells Us*. New York: Guilford Press.

2. American Psychiatric Association. (2000). *Diagnostic and Statistical Manual of Mental Disorders, 4th Edition (DSM-IV)*. Washington, DC: Author.

3. Kessler, R.C., Adler L., Barkley R., et al. (2006). The prevalence and correlates of adult ADHD in the United States: Results from the National Comorbidity Survey Replication. *American Journal of Psychiatry, 163,* 716–723.

4. US Census Bureau. United States Census 2000. U.S. Summary. July 2002.

5. Biederman, J., Faraone, S.V., et al. (2006). Functional impairments in adults with self reports of diagnosed ADHD: A controlled study of 1001 adults in the community. *Journal of Clinical Psychiatry, 67*(4), 524–540.

6. Biederman, J., and Faraone, S.V. (2006). The effects of attention-deficit/hyperactivity disorder on employment and household income. *Medscape General Medicine, 8*(3), 12.

7. de Graff, R., Kessler, R.C., Fayyad, J., et al. (2008). The prevalence and effects of attention-deficit/hyperactivity disorder (ADHD) on the performance of workers: Results from the WHO World Mental Health Survey Initiative. *Occupational Environmental Medicine, 65,* 835–842.

8. Biederman, J., Faraone, S.V., Spencer, T., Wilens, T., Norman, D., Lapey, K.A., et al. (1993). Patterns of psychiatric comorbidity, cognition, and psychosocial functioning in adults with attention deficit hyperactivity disorder. *American Journal of Psychiatry, 150,* 1792–1798.

9. Fischer, M., Barkley, R.A., Edelbrock, C.S., and Smallish, L. (1990). The adolescent outcome of hyperactive children diagnosed by research criteria: II. Academic, attentional, and neuropsychological status. *Journal of Consulting and Clinical Psychology, 58*(5), 580–588.

10. De Quiros, G.B., and Kinsbourne, M. (2001). Adult ADHD: Analysis of self-ratings on a behavior questionnaire. In J.Wasserstein, L. Wolf, and F. Lefever (Eds.), *Adult attention deficit disorder: Brain mechanisms and life outcomes. Annals of the New York Academy of Sciences, 931,* 140–147.

11. Biederman, J., Faraone, S.V., Keenan, K., et al. (1992). Further evidence for family-genetic risk factors in attention deficit hyperactivity disorder. Patterns of comorbidity in probands and relatives psychiatrically and pediatrically referred samples. *Archives of General Psychiatry, 49*(9), 728–738.

12. Minde, K., Eakin, L., Hechtman, L., et al. (2003). The psychosocial functioning of children and spouses of adults with ADHD. *Journal of Child Psychology and Psychiatry, 44*(4), 637–646.

13. Barkley, R. A. (2006). *Attention Deficit Hyperactivity Disorder: A Handbook for Diagnosis and Treatment* (3rd ed.). New York: Guilford Press.

14. Barkley, R.A., Fischer, M., Smallish L., and Fletcher K. (2006). Young adult follow-up of hyperactive children: Adaptive functioning in major life activities. *Journal of the American Academy of Child and Adolescent Psychiatry, 45,* 192–202.

15. Szatmari, P., Offord, D.R., and Boyle, M.H. (1989). Ontario Child Health Study: Prevalence of Attention Deficit Disorder with Hyperactivity. *Journal of Child Psychology and Psychiatry, 30*(2), 219–223.

16. Faraone, S.V., Biederman, J., Lehman, B.K., Keenan, K., Norman, D., Seidman, L.J., et al. (1993). Evidence for the independent familial transmission of attention deficit hyper-activity disorder and learning disabilities: Results from a family genetic study. *American Journal of Psychiatry, 150,* 891–895

17. Barkley, R.A., Fischer, M., Edelbrock, C.S., et al. (1990). The adolescent outcome of hyperactive children diagnosed by research criteria: I. An 8-year prospective follow-up study. *Journal of the American Academy of Child & Adolescent Psychiatry, 29*(4), 546–557.

18. Barkley, R.A., DuPaul, G.J., and McMurray, M.B. (1990). Comprehensive evaluation of attention deficit disorder with and without hyperactivity as defined by research criteria. *Journal of Consulting and Clinical Psychology, 58*(6), 775–789

19. Barkley, R.A., Fischer, M., Smallish ,L., et al. (2004). Young adult follow-up of hyperactive children: Antisocial activities and drug use. *Journal of Child Psychology and Psychiatry, 45,* 195–211.

20. Rapaport, M.D., Scanlan, S.W., and Denney, C.B. (1999). Attention-deficit/hyperactivity disorder and scholastic achievement: A model of dual developmental pathways. *The Journal of Child Psychology and Psychiatry and Allied Disciplines, 40,* 1169–1183.

21. Barkley, R.A., Murphy, K.R., and Kwasnik D. (1996). Psychological adjustment and adaptive impairments in young adults with ADHD. *Journal of Attention Disorders, 1,* 41–54.

22. Murphy, K.R., Barkley, R.A., and Bush, T. (1996). Young adults with ADHD: Subtype differences in comorbidities and adaptive impairments. *Comprehensive Psychiatry, 37,* 393–401.

23. Murphy, K.R., Barkley R.A., and Bush, T. (2002). Young adults with ADHD: Subtype differences in comorbidity, educational, and clinical history. *Journal of Nervous and Mental Disease, 190,* 147–157.

24. Werner, E., Bierman, J., French, F., et al. (1968). Reproductive and environmental casualties: a report of the 10-year follow-up of the children of the Kauai pregnancy study. *Pediatrics, 42*(1), 112–127.

25. Weiss, G., and Hechtman, L. (1993). *Hyperactive Children Grown Up: ADHD in Children, Adolescents, and Adults.* New York: Guilford Press.

26. Weiss, G., Hechtman, L., Perlman, T., Hopkins, J., & Wener, A. (1979). Hyperactives as young adults: A controlled prospective ten-year follow-up of 75 children. *Archives of General Psychiatry, 36,* 675–681.

27. Richards, T.L., Deffenbacher, J.L., Rosen, L.A., et al. (2006). Driving anger and driving behavior in adults with ADHD. *Journal of Attention Disorders, 10,* 54–64.

28. Knouse, L., Bagwell, C.L., Barkley, R.A., et al. (2005). Accuracy of self-evaluation in adults with ADHD. *Journal of Attention Disorders, 8*(4), 221–234.

29. Barkley, R.A. (2004). Driving impairments in teens and adults with attention-deficit/hyperactivity disorder. *Psychiatric Clinics of North America, 27,* 233–260.

30. Barkley, R.A., Guevremont, D.G., Anastopoulor, A.D., Dupaul, G.J., and Selton, T.L. (1993). Driving related risks and outcome of attention-deficit/hyperactivity disorder in adolescents and young adults: A 3–5 year follow-up survey. *Pediatrics, 92,* 212–218.

31. Barkley, R.A., Murphy, K.R., DuPaul, G.J., and Bush, T. (2002). Driving in young adults with attention deficit hyperactivity disorder: Knowledge, performance, adverse outcomes, and the role of executive functioning. *Journal of the International Neuropsychology Society, 8,* 655–672.

32. Barkley, R.A., Murphy, K.R., O'Connell, T., Anderson, D., and Connor, D.F. (2006). Effects of two doses of alcohol on simulator driving performance in adults with attention-deficit/hyperactivity disorder. *Neuropsychology, 20*(1), 77–87.

33. Cox, D.J., Merkel, R.L., Davatchev, B. et al. (2000). Effect of stimulant medication on driving performance of young adults with attention-deficit hyperactivity disorder: A preliminary double-blind placebo controlled trial. *Journal of Nervous and Mental Disease, 188,* 230–234.

34. Cox, D.J., Punja, M., Powers, K., et al. (2006). Manual transmission enhances attention and driving performance of ADHD adolescent males. *Journal of Attention Disorders, 10*(2), 212–216.

35. Biederman, J., Wilens, T., Mick, E., et. al. (1991). Pharmacotherapy of attention-deficit/hyperactivity disorder reduces risk for substance use disorder. *Pediatrics, 104*(2), e20.

36. Barkley, R.A. (1997). *ADHD and the Nature of Self-Control.* New York: Guilford Press.

37. Adler, L., and Cohen, J. (2004). Diagnosis and evaluation of adults with attention-deficit/hyperactivity disorder. *Psychiatric Clinics of North America, 27,* 187–201.

38. Conners, C.K., Erhardt, D., Epstein, J.N., et al. (1999). Self-ratings of ADHD symptoms in adults: I. Factor and normative data. *Journal of Attention Disorders, 3*(3), 141–151.

39. Nigg, J.T. (2006). *What Causes ADHD? Understanding What Goes Wrong and Why.* New York: Guilford Press.

40. Comings, D.E. (2001). Clinical and molecular genetics of ADHD and Tourette Syndrome: Two related polygenic disorders. *Annals of the New York Academy of Sciences, 931,* 50–83

41. Biederman, J., Faraone, S.V., Mick E., et al. (1995). High risk for attention deficit hyperactivity disorder among children of parents with childhood onset of the disorder: A pilot study. *American Journal of Psychiatry, 152,* 431–435.

42. Bush, G., Frazier, J.A., Rauch, S.L., et al. (1999). Anterior cingulate cortex dysfunction in attention-deficit/hyperactivity disorder revealed by fMRI and the counting stroop. *Biological Psychiatry, 45,* 1542–52.

43. Williams, Z.M., Bush, G., Rauch, S.L., Cosgrove, G.R., and Eskandar, E.N. (2004). Human anterior cingulated neurons and the integration of monetary reward with motor responses. *Nature Reviews Neuroscience, 7,* 1370–1375.

44. Castellanos, F.X., Lee, P.P., Sharp, W., et al. (2002). Developmental trajectories of brain volume abnormalities in children and adolescents with attention-deficit/hyperactivity disorder. *Journal of the American Medical Association, 288,* 1740–1748.

45. Tzelepis, A., Schubiner, H., and Warbasse, L.H. (1995). Differential diagnosis and psychiatric comorbidity patterns in adult attention deficit disorder. In K. Nadeau (Ed). *A comprehensive guide to attention deficit disorder in adults: Research, diagnosis, treatment* (pp. 35–37). New York: Brunner/Mazel.

46. Roy-Byrne, P., Scheele, L., Brinkley, J. et al. (1997). Adult attention-deficit hyperactivity disorder: Assessment guidelines based on clinical presentation to a specialty clinic. *Comprehensive Psychiatry, 38*, 133–140.

47. Applegate, B., Lahey, B.B., Hart, E.L., et al. (1997). Validity of the age of onset criterion for ADHD: A report from the DSM-IV field trials. *Journal of the American Academy of Child and Adolescent Psychiatry, 36*, 1211–1121.

48. Murphy, K.R., and Barkley, R.A. (1996). Prevalence of DSM-IV ADHD symptoms in adult licensed drivers. *Journal of Attention Disorders, 1*, 147–161.

49. Nigg, J.T., Stavro, G., Ettenhofer, M., Hambrick, D., Miller, T., and Henderson, J.M. (2005). Executive functions and ADHD in adults: Evidence for selective effects on ADHD symptom domains. *Journal of Abnormal Psychology, 114*, 706–717.

50. Americans with Disabilities Act of 1990. Available online at: http://www.ada.gov/pubs/ada.htm.

51. Wilens, T.E. (2004). Attention-deficit/hyperactivity disorder and the substance use disorders: The nature of their relationship, subtypes at risk, and treatment issues. *Psychiatric Clinics of North America, 27*(2), 283–301.

52. Selzer, M.L. (1971). The Michigan Alcoholism Screening Test (MAST): The quest for a new diagnostic instrument. *American Journal of Psychiatry, 127*, 1653–1658.

53. Wender, P.H. (1995). *Attention-deficit hyperactivity disorder in adults.* New York: Oxford University Press.

54. Barkley, R.A., and Murphy, K.R. (2006). *Attention Deficit Hyperactivity Disorder: A Clinical Workbook* (3rd ed.). New York: Guilford Press

55. Barkley, R.A. (2007). *Barkley's Quick-Check for Adult ADHD Diagnosis.* Sudbury, MA: Jones and Bartlett.

56. First, M.B., Spitzer, R.L., Gibbon, M., and Williams, J.B.W. (2002). *Structured Clinical Interview for DSM-IV-TR Axis I Disorders, Research Version, Non-patient Edition. (SCID-I/NP).* New York: Biometrics Research, New York State Psychiatric Institute.

57. Kessler, R.C., Adler, L., Ames, M., Demler, O., Faraone, S., Hiripi, E., et al. (2005). The World Health Organization Adult ADHD Self-Report Scale (ASRS). *Psychological Medicine, 35*(2), 245–256.

58. Spencer, T., and Adler, L. (2004). Diagnostic approaches to adult attention-deficit/hyperactivity disorder. *Primary Psychiatry, 11*, 49–53.

59. DuPaul, G.J., Power, T.J., Anastopoulos, A.D., et al. (1998). *ADHD Rating Scale-IV: Checklists, Norms, and Clinical Interpretation.* New York: Guilford Press.

60. Spencer, T., Adler, L., Biederman, J., et al. (2007, May). *Use of the Adult ADHD Investigator Symptom Rating Scale (AISRS) as an instrument to measure the impact of methylphenidate therapy on adult signs and symptoms of ADHD.* Paper presented at the annual meeting of the American Psychiatric Association, San Diego, CA.

61. Barkley, R.A. (2007). *Barkley's Adult ADHD Quick Screen.* Sudbury, MA: Jones and Bartlett.

62. Brown, T.E.(2001). *Brown Attention-Deficit Disorder Scales®.* San Antonio, TX: PsychCorp.

63. Conners, C.K., Erhardt, D., Parker, J.D.A., et al. (1998). *The Conners Adult ADHD Rating Scale (CAARS)*. Toronto: Multi-Health Systems, Inc.

64. Derogatis, L.R. (1994). *Symptom Checklist-90-Revised (SCL-90-R®)*. CITY: National Computer Systems, Inc.

65. Gioia, G.A., Isquith, P.K., Guy, S.C., and Kenworthy, L. (2000). *BRIEF: Behavior Rating Inventory of Executive Function*. Odessa, FL: Psychological Assessment Resources, Inc.

66. Roth, R.M., Isquith, P.K., and Gioia, G.A. (2005). *BRIEF-A: Behavioral Rating Inventory of Executive Functions – Adult Version*. Lutz, FL: Psychological Assessment Resources.

67. Conners, C. K. (1995). *The Conners Continuous Performance Test*. North Tonawanda, NY: Multi-Health Systems.

68. Epstein, J.N., Conners, C.K., Sitarenios, G., and Erhardt, D. (1998). Continuous performance test results of adults with attention deficit hyperactivity disorder. *The Clinical Neuropsychologist, 12*, 155–168.

69. Schopick, D. (1998). *Highly Effective Approaches to Making the Conners' CPT Work in Your Clinical Practice*. North Tonawanda, NY: Multi-Health Systems, Inc.

70. Stroop, J.P. (1935). Studies of interference in serial verbal reactions. *Journal of Experimental Psychology, 18*, 643–662.

71. Wechsler, D. (2008). *Manual for the Wechsler Adult Intelligence Test, Fourth Edition. (WAIS-IV)*. San Antonio, TX: Psychological Corp.

72. Zametkin, A.J., and Rapoport, J.L. (1987). Neurobiology of attention deficit disorder with hyperactivity: Where have we come in 50 years? *Journal of the American Academy of Child and Adolescent Psychiatry, 26*, 676–686.

73. Pliszka, S.R., Crismon, M.L., Hughes, C.W., et al. (2007). CMAP ADHD and comorbid aggression algorithm. *Journal of the American Academy of Child & Adolescent Psychiatry, 46*(1), 2–3.

74. Bradley, C. (1937). The behaviour of children receiving benzedrine. *American Journal of Psychiatry, 94*, 577–585.

75. Biederman, J., and Spencer, T.J. (2004). Psychopharmarcology of adults with attention-deficit/hyperactivity disorder. *Primary Psychiatry, 11*(7), 57–62.

76. Goodman, D. (2006). Treatment and assessment of ADHD in adults. In J. Biederman, (Ed.), *ADHD Across the Life Span: From Research to Clinical Practice—An Evidence-Based Understanding*. Hasbrouck Heights, NJ: Veritas Institute for Medical Education, Inc.

77. Mattes, J.A., Boswell, L., et al. (1984). Methylphenidate effects on symptoms of attention deficit disorder in adults. *Archives of General Psychiatry, 41*, 1059–1063.

78. Spencer, T., Wilens, T.E., et al. (1995). A double blind, crossover comparison of methylphenidate and placebo in adults with childhood onset attention deficit hyperactivity disorder. *Archives of General Psychiatry, 52*, 434–443.

79. Wender, P.H., Reimherr, F.W., et al. (1985). A controlled study of methylphenidate in the treatment of attention deficit disorder, residual type, in adults. *American Journal of Psychiatry, 142*, 547–552.

80. Iaboni, F., Bouffard, R., Minde, K., et al. (1996). The efficacy of methylphenidate in treating adults with attention-deficit/hyperactivity disorder. *Scientific Proceedings of the American Academy of Child and Adolescent Psychiatry.* Philadelphia, PA: American Academy of Child and Adolescent Psychiatry.

81. Ratey, J., Greenberg, M., et al. (1991). Combination of treatments for attention deficit disorders in adults. *Journal of Nervous and Mental Disease, 176,* 699–701.

82. Focalin [tablets package insert (T2001-85)]. East Hanover, NJ: Novartis Pharmaceuticals Corp.

83. Vyvanse™ [tablets package insert]. Wayne, PA: Shire US Inc.

84. Biederman, J., Hodgkins, P., Krishnan, S., and Findling, R.L. (2007). Efficacy and tolerability of lisdexamfetamine (NRP104) in children with attention-deficit/hyperacticity disorder (ADHD): A phase 3, randomized, multi-center, randomized, double-blind, forced-dose, parallel group study. *Clinical Therapeutics, 29,* 450–463.

85. Schuster, C.R. (2006). History and current perspectives on the use of drug formulations to decrease the abuse of prescription drugs. *Drug Alcohol Dependence, 83,* S8–S14.

86. Guy, W. (1976). *Clinical global impressions. ECDEU assessment manual for psychopharmacology.* Rockville, MD: US Department of Health, Education and Welfare.

87. Adler, L., Goodman, D., Kollins, A.H., Weisler, R.H., Krishman, S., Zhang, Y., et al. (2008). Double-blind, placebo-controlled study of the efficacy and safety of lisdexamfetamine dimesylate in adult with attention-deficit/hyperactivity disorder. *Journal of Clinical Psychology, 69,* 1364–1373.

88. Adler, L., Goodman, D., Kollins, A.H., et al. (2008). Double-blind, placebo-controlled study of the efficacy and safety of lisdexamfetamine dimesylate in adults with attention-deficit/hyperactivity disorder. *Journal of Clinical Psychiatry, 69,* 1364–1373.

89. Adler, L., et al. (2007, October 25). *Efficacy and safety of lisdexamfetamine dimesylate in adults with attention deficit hyperactivity disorder.* Paper presented at the annual meeting of the American Academy of Child and Adolescent Psychiatry, Boston, MA.

90. Concerta [tablets package insert (0011791-1 PPI)]. Fort Washington, PA: McNeil Consumer Healthcare.

91. Medori, R., Ramos-Quiroga, A., Casas, M., Kooiji, J.J.S., Niemla, A., Trott, G.E., et al. (2008). A randomized, placebo-controlled trial of three fixed dosages of prolonged-release OROS methylphenidate in adults with attention-deficit/hyperactivity disorder. *Biological Psychiatry, 63,* 981–989.

92. Adderall XR [package insert (403952)]. Florence, KY: Shire US Inc.

93. Strattera [package insert (PV 3750AMP)]. Indianapolis, IN: Eli Lilly & Company.

94. Michelson, D., Adler, L., Spencer, T., et al. (2003). Atomoxetine in adults with ADHD: Two randomized, placebo-controlled studies. *Biologcial Psychiatry, 53*(2), 112–120.

95. Wilens, T., Prince, J., et al. (2001). *An open study of sustained-release bupropion in adults with ADHD and substance use disorders.* Paper presented at the annual meeting of AACAP, Honolulu, HI.

96. Davis, W.B., Bentivoglio, P., et al. (2001). Bupropion sustained release in adolescents with comorbid attention-deficit/hyperactivity disorder and depression. *Journal of the American Academy of Child and Adolescent Psychiatry, 40*(3), 307–314.

97. Newcorn, J., and Weiss, M.D. (2006, April). *Adult ADHD: Effective Treatment Strategies (online CME)*. Based on Adult ADHD Academic Council monograph.

98. Goodman, D.W. (2007). Adult ADHD: Diagnosis and treatment in the presence of comorbid depression. *Psychiatric Times CME, Suppl*, 5–8.

99. Levin, F.R., Evans, S.M., et al. (2006). Treatment of methadone-maintained patients with adult ADHD: Double-blind comparison of methylphenidate, bupropion and placebo. *Drug and Alcohol Dependence, 81*(2), 137–148.

100. Levin, F.R., Evans, S.M., et al. (1999). Practical guidelines for the treament of substance abusers with adult attention-deficit hyperactivity disorder. *Psychiatric Services, 50*(8), 1001–1003.

101. Brown, T.E. (2004). Atomoxetine and stimulants in combination for treatment of attention deficit hyperactivity disorder: Four case reports. *Journal of Child and Adolescent Psychopharmacology, 14*(1), 129–136.

102. MTA Cooperative Group. (1999). A fourteen month randomized clinical trial of treatment strategies for attention deficit hyperactivity disorder. *Archives of General Psychiatry, 56,* 1073–1086.

103. Conners, C.K., and Erhardt, D., (1998). Attention-deficit hyperactivity disorder in children and adolescents, In M. Herson and A. Bellack (Eds.), *Children and Adolescents: Clinical Formulation and Treatment*. New York: Elsevier Science.

104. Spencer, T., Biederman, J., Wilens, T., Harding, J. O'Donnell, D, and Griffen, S. (1996). Pharmacotherapy of attention-deficit hyperactivity disorder across the life cycle. *Journal of the American Academy of Child and Adolescent Psychiatry, 355*, 409–432.

105. Safren, S.A., Sprich, S., Chulvik, S., et al. (2004). Psychosocial treatments for adults with attention-deficit/hyperactivity disorder. *Psychiatric Clinics of North America, 27,* 349–360.

106. Murphy, K.R. (2006). Counseling the adult with ADHD. In Barkley R.A. (Ed.), *Attention deficit hyperactivity disorder: A handbook for diagnosis and treatment* (3rd ed.). New York: Guilford Press.

107. Safren, S.A. (2006). Cognitive Behavioral Approaches to ADHD Treatment in Adulthood. *Journal of Clinical Psychiatry, 67*(8), 46–50.

108. Kohlberg, J., and Nadeau, K. (2002). *ADD-friendly ways to organize your life*. New York: Brunner-Routledge.

109. Beck, A. (1995). *Cognitive Therapy: Basics and Beyond*. New York: Guilford Press.

110. Stevenson, C.S., Whitmont, S., Bomholt, L., et al. (2002). A cognitive remediation programme for adults with attention deficit hyperactivity disorder. *Australian and New Zealand Journal of Psychiatry, 36,* 610–616.

111. Weiss, M., Hectman, L., et al. (1999). *ADHD in Adulthood: A guide to current theory, diagnosis, and treatment*. Baltimore, MD: The Johns Hopkins University Press.

Index

A

Adderall® XR, 39, 41, 42, 44
ADHD. *See also* Adolescents with ADHD; Adults
    with ADHD; Children with ADHD
        across lifespan, 9–12
        causes of, 4, 12–14
        educational achievement and, 5–6, 52, 61–62
        explanation of, 1
        intelligence and, 6
        neurobiology of, 12–13
        neurotransmitters in, 13, 38, 42
ADHD Clinical Diagnostic Scale (ACDS), 3
ADHD in Adults: What the Science Says (National
    Institute of Mental Health), 2
ADHD Rating Scale (ADHD-RS), 3
Adolescents with ADHD
        characteristics of, 10, 11
        educational achievement for, 61–62
        neurobiology of, 12–13
        stimulants for, 39
        suicidal ideation and, 43
Adult ADHD Interview, 30
*Adult ADHD Investigator Symptom Rating Scale
    (AISRS)*, 31
Adult ADHD Self-Report Scale (ASRS), 31
Adults with ADHD
        across lifespan, 9–12
        age of onset of, 18–19, 24
        characteristics of, 1–2, 10
        child-rearing by, 60
        diagnostic criteria for, 18–20
        driving safety and, 8–9, 65
        educational achievement and, 5–6, 52, 61–62
        employment issues and, 6–7, 62–64
        executive functions in, 11, 13, 20, 23, 33, 38, 52
        health and lifestyle problems in, 3–4, 59
        high-risk behavior in, 4
        money management and, 8, 64
        neurotransmitters in, 13, 38, 42
        psychosocial treatment for, 37, 49, 51–58
        relationship problems in, 4–5, 57–58, 60
        sexual health of, 59
        statistics related to, 1, 7
        symptom patterns in, 1, 17, 19–20
        working memory in, 11, 13, 20
Age
        of ADHD onset, 18–19, 24
        symptom patterns and, 1
American Academy of Child and Adolescent
    Psychiatry (AACAP), 39
Americans with Disabilities Act (ADA), 20, 62
Amphetamines, 38–42, 44, 48. *See also* Stimulant
    medications
Anhedonia, 28

Antidepressant medications, 43, 48
Anxiety disorders, 25, 28, 46
Archival records, 32
Assessment. *See also* Diagnosis; Diagnostic criteria;
    specific tests
        age role in, 1–3, 18–19
        archival records and, 30, 32
        interviews and, 19, 30
        neuropsychological tests and, 30, 33–34
        self-reporting scales, 19, 30, 31–32, 41–42
        tools for, 30
Atomoxetine, 13, 39, 42–45, 47, 48
Attention deficit/hyperactivity disorder (ADHD). *See*
    ADHD; Adult ADHD
Automobile safety, 8–9

B

Barkley's Adult ADHD Quick Screen, 31
Barkley's Quick Check for Adult ADHD Diagnosis, 30
Basal ganglia, 12
Behavioral therapy. *See* Cognitive-behavioral therapy
    (CBT)
*Behavior Rating Inventory of Executive Function
    (BRIEF)*, 33
Benedrine, 39
Bipolar disorder (BPD), 25, 26
Borderline personality disorder, 28
Brain development/function, 12–13
Brown ADD Rating Scale, 31
Bupropion, 43, 48

C

Causes of ADHD
        environmental biohazards as, 12
        genetics as, 4, 12, 14
        neurobiology and, 12–14
Child-rearing, 60
Children with ADHD
        of ADHD parents, 4–5
        anxiety disorders in, 28
        characteristics of, 10
        comorbid conditions in, 29
        educational achievement of, 5–6
        genetics and, 12
        neurobiology of, 12–13
        stimulants for, 39
        suicidal ideation and, 43
Clinical Global Impressions-Improvement scale
    (CGI-I), 41
Cognitive-behavioral therapy (CBT), 37, 49, 51,
    54–56
College education, 61–62
Comorbid conditions
        anxiety as, 25, 28, 246

depression as, 2, 4, 17, 24–28, 56, 59
explanation of, 2, 29
proper treatment of, 17
stimulants and, 46
substance abuse/dependence as, 27
Composit International Diagnostic Interview (CIDI), 3
Concerta®, 38, 39, 41, 44
Conners' Adult Attention-Deficit Rating Scale (CAARS), 31, 41, 42
Conners' Continuous Performance Test (CPT), 33
Couples therapy, 57–58

D

Depression, 2, 4, 17, 24–28, 56, 59
Desipramine, 43, 48
Dexmethylphenidate, 39, 40, 44
Diagnosis. *See also* Assessment
challenges related to, 21–22
differential, 24–25
malingering, 22
threshold for, 20
under-reporting of impairment and, 22
Diagnostic and Statistical Manual of Mental Disorders, Fourth Edition, Text Revision (DSM-IV-TR) (American Psychiatric Association), 15–20
Diagnostic criteria
for adult patients, 18–20
anxiety disorders and, 28
bipolar disorder and, 26
borderline personality disorder and, 28
comorbitidy and, 29
depression and, 27–28
differential diagnosis and, 24–25
in *DSM-IV-TR*, 15–20
new symptom list as, 23
overview of current, 15, 16
substance use/abuse and, 27
Differential diagnosis, 24–25
Distractibility, 8, 56
Dopamine, 13–14, 38, 42
Dorsal lateral prefrontal area, 38
Driving safety, 8–9, 65
DSM-IV ADHD Rating Scale, 40–42
DSM-IV-TR. See Diagnostic and Statistical Manual of Mental Disorders, Fourth Edition, Text Revision (DSM-IV-TR) (American Psychiatric Association)

E

Education, patient, 49
Educational achievement, 5–6, 52, 61–62
Employment issues, 6–7, 62–64
Executive functioning, 11, 13, 20, 23, 33, 38, 52
Extended-release medications, 39–42

F

FDA-approved medications, 39–41, 43, 44, 48

Finances, 64
First-line medications, 39, 48
Focalin™ XR, 39–41, 44
Frontal lobe, 12

G

Genetics, 4, 12, 14
Group therapy, 58

H

Hyperactivity, 1, 2, 5, 13, 15–16, 20–21, 26

I

Immediate-release medications, 38
Impairment, 20–21
Impulsivity, 1, 3, 5, 8, 13, 15–17, 20–21, 26, 54
Inattention, 1, 3, 5, 9, 11, 13, 15–16, 20–21, 24, 26
Inhibition, 20, 21, 24
Inhibitory effects, 38
Intelligence, 6
Interviews
assessment, 19, 30
diagnostic, 3
structured, 30
Intra-person discrepancy standard, 20, 21

L

Lifestyle problems, 3–4
Lisdexamfetamine dimesylate, 40–41, 44

M

Malingering, 21, 22
Medical College of Wisconsin Study in Milwaukee (Milwaukee study), 2, 9, 22, 23, 29
Medications. *See also specific medications*
amphetamines as, 38–42, 44, 48
antidepressants as, 43, 48
atomoxetine, 13, 39, 42–45, 47, 48
comorbid conditions and, 46, 47
dexmethylphenidate, 39, 40, 44
extended-release, 39–42
FDA-approved, 39–41, 43, 44, 48
first-line, 39, 48
immediate-release, 38
lisdexamfetamine dimesylate, 40–41, 44
management of, 46, 48
methylphenidate, 38, 39, 41, 44
mixed amphetamine salts, 39, 41–42, 44
nonstimulant, 42–44
off-label use of, 37–40
selective norepinephrine reuptake inhibitor, 13, 42
side effects of, 46, 47
stimulant, 13, 38–42, 44–45
treatment goals for, 48–49
vital signs and, 40

Memory, 11, 13, 20
Mentors, 63
Mesostriatal pathway, 38
Methylphenidate (MPH), 38, 39, 41, 44
Michigan Alcohol Screening Test, 27
Mixed amphetamine salts (MAS), 39, 41–42, 44. *See also* Stimulant medications
Money management, 8, 64
Multimodal Treatment of ADHD Study (MTA), 51

N

National Institute of Mental Health (NIMH), 2
Neuropsychiatric disorders, 1
Neuropsychological tests
    Behavior Rating Inventory of Executive Function, 33
    Conners' Continuous Performance Test, 33
    Stroop Word Color Test, 34
    Wechsler Adult Intelligence Test, Fourth Edition - Digit Span Subtest, 34
Neurotransmitters, 13, 38, 42
Nigrostriatal pathway, 38
Nonstimulant medications, 42–44
Norepinephrine, 13, 14, 38, 39, 42, 43

O

Off-label use of medication, 37–40
Organization skills, 23, 55, 56
Osmotic release oral system (OROS), 41

P

Panic attacks, 25
Patient education, 49
Personal coaching, 62
Pharmacological treatment. *See* Medications
Post-Traumatic Stress Disorder (PTSD), 25
Prodrug, 40
Psychiatric disorders, 25, 26, 46
Psychoeducation, 53–54
Psychosocial treatment of adult ADHD
    cognitive-behavioral therapy as, 37, 49, 51, 54–56
    couples therapy as, 57–58
    goals of, 51–52
    group therapy as, 58
    patient and family education, 51, 52
    psychoeducation as, 53–54
    support person as, 57

R

Rating scales. *See also* Self-reporting scales
    ADHD Clinical Diagnostic Scale, 3
    ADHD Rating Scale, 3
    Clinical Global Impressions-Improvement scale, 41
    Composit International Diagnostic Interview, 3
    DSM-IV ADHD, 40–42

WHO-Disability Assessment Scale, 3
WHO Health and Work Performance Questionnaire, 3
Relationship problems, 4–5, 57–58, 60
Research. *See also specific studies*
    Medical College of Wisconsin Study in Milwaukee, 2, 9, 22, 23, 29
    overview of, 1–2
    twin studies and, 12
    UMass Study and, 2, 5, 8, 20, 22, 23, 29

S

Safety, automobile, 8–9, 65
Selective norepinephrine reuptake inhibitor (SNRI), 13, 14, 42
Self-control, 1, 9, 11, 17
Self-esteem, 28, 52
Self-image, 53
Self-reporting scales. *See also* Rating scales
    Adult ADHD Investigator Symptom Rating Scale, 31
    Adult ADHD Self-Report Scale, 31
    Barkley's Adult ADHD Quick Screen, 31
    Brown ADD Rating Scale, 31
    Conners' Adult Attention-Deficit Rating Scale, 31, 41– 42
    Symptom Checklist 90-Revised, 32
    Wender Utah Rating Scale, 32
Sleep difficulties, 28
Specialized peer-group standard, 20, 21
Stimulant medications. *See also* Medications; *specific medications*
    benefits of, 13, 38
    for children, 39
    comorbid conditions and, 46
    contraindications and adverse events associated with, 45
    descriptions of specific, 40–42
    long- vs. short-acting, 44–45, 48
    misuse and abuse of, 45
    side effects of, 47
Strattera®, 39, 42–44, 47
Stress, 24–25
Stroop Word Color Test, 34
Structured Clinical Interview for DSM-IV (SCID), 30
Structured interviews, 30
Substance abuse, 27, 45, 46
Suicidal ideation, 43
Support persons, 57
Symptom Checklist 90-Revised, 32

T

Teratogens, 12
Texas Treatment Algorithm, 46
Therapy. *See also* Psychosocial treatment of adult ADHD
    cognitive-behavioral, 37, 49, 51, 54–56

couples, 57–58
group, 58
Time management, 1, 3, 17, 54, 55
Treatment. *See* Cognitive-behavioral therapy (CBT); Medications; Psychosocial treatment
Tricyclic antidepressants (TCAs), 42, 43
Twin studies, 12

U

University of Massachusetts Medical School (UMass Study), 2, 5, 8, 20, 22, 23, 29

V

Vital signs, 40
Vocational counseling, 63

Vocational training, 61–62
Vyvanse™, 39–41, 44

W

Wechsler Adult Intelligence Test, Fourth Edition (WAIS-IV)-Digit Span Subtest, 34
Wender Utah Rating Scale (WURS), 32
WHO-Disability Assessment Scale, 3
WHO Health and Work Performance Questionnaire, 3
Working memory, 11, 13, 20
World Health Organization (WHO), 2–3, 7